5.50

Mid-century Psychiatry

Mid-century Psychiatry

——AN OVERVIEW——

EDITED BY

ROY R. GRINKER, M.D.

*Director of Institute for
Psychosomatic and Psychiatric Research and Training
Michael Reese Hospital
Chicago, Illinois*

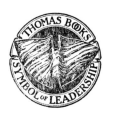

CHARLES C THOMAS · PUBLISHER
Springfield · Illinois · U.S.A.

CHARLES C THOMAS • PUBLISHER
BANNERSTONE HOUSE
301–327 East Lawrence Avenue, Springfield, Illinois, U.S.A.

Published simultaneously in the British Commonwealth of Nations by
BLACKWELL SCIENTIFIC PUBLICATIONS, LTD., OXFORD, ENGLAND

Published simultaneously in Canada by
THE RYERSON PRESS, TORONTO

Printed in the United States of America

CONTRIBUTORS

Roy R. Grinker, M.D. *Director, Institute for Psychosomatic and Psychiatric Research and Training, Michael Reese Hospital; Clinical Professor of Psychiatry, University of Illinois, College of Medicine.*

Percival Bailey, Ph.D., M.D. *Professor of Neurology and Neurosurgery, University of Illinois College of Medicine, Director, Illinois Psychopathic Laboratory.*

Ralph W. Gerard, Ph.D., M.D. *Professor of Physiology, University of Illinois, College of Medicine.*

George L. Engel, M.D. *Associate Professor of Psychiatry and Medicine, University of Rochester Medical and Dental School.*

Therese Benedek, M.D. *Staff Member, Chicago Psychoanalytic Institute.*

David Shakow, Ph.D. *Professor of Psychology, University of Illinois College of Medicine.*

Howard S. Liddell, Ph.D. *Professor of Experimental Psychology, Cornell University Medical School.*

David M. Levy, M.D. *Professor of Psychoanalysis, Columbia University Medical School.*

M. Ralph Kaufman, M.D. *Chairman, Department of Psychiatry, Mount Sinai Hospital, New York; Professor of Psychiatry, Columbia University Medical School.*

Thomas M. French, M.D. *Associate Director, Chicago Psychoanalytic Institute.*

Charles S. Johnson, Ph.D. *President, Fiske University.*

Franz Alexander, M.D. *Director, Chicago Psychoanalytic Institute; Clinical Professor of Psychiatry, University of Illinois, College of Medicine.*

John P. Spiegel, M.D. *Associate Director, Institute for Psychosomatic and Psychiatric Research and Training, Michael Reese Hospital.*

v

PREFACE

On June 1, 1951, the Institute for Psychosomatic and Psychiatric Research and Training of the Michael Reese Hospital was dedicated by a gathering of scientists who spoke on varying aspects of *Mid-century Psychiatry*. Their contributions are recorded as contemporary statements and promises of several disciplines that have contributed greatly to the science of behavior. This symposium, far from indicating that the twentieth mid-century was close to producing the awaited synthesis of many disciplines into a behavioral science, emphasized the absence of a basic or unitary concept of human nature, the polyglot nature of interdisciplinary communications and the failure of diverse and multileveled operational procedures to permit sound correlations. Yet today there are many signs to indicate that these goals are understood with greater clarity and that many are engaged in positive efforts to attain them despite huge obstacles.

I am deeply indebted to the participants of our dedicatory exercises for their labors in producing these contributions, for the time and effort they spent in presenting their material and for permission to include their work in this volume.

Roy R. Grinker, M.D.

Chicago, Illinois
July 1, 1951

CONTENTS

M*id-century* P*sychiatry*

INTRODUCTION

By
Roy R. Grinker[*]

With this dedication and formal opening of the Institute for Psychosomatic and Psychiatric Research and Training, after long planning, a new phase in psychiatry now begins at Michael Reese Hospital and in the community of Chicago. Another forward step has been taken by an institution which has pioneered many aspects of medical progress since its founding, including the acceptance and development of dynamic psychiatry for over thirty years.

Thirty-three years ago Mr. Sidney Schwarz, who has ever been a stimulation and guiding spirit of psychiatry in this community, prevailed upon a group of staff doctors of various specialties to discuss the over-all problems of indigent patients who seemed to fit into a single category. These patients were elderly males whose life patterns were replete with failure, domestic difficulties, alcoholism and varying degrees of delinquency and who ended their sordid roles in ward beds anxiously gasping with cardiac decompensation for more unhappy days. The professional group in conferences considered these patterns of living, recognized the typical personality profiles and hopelessly abandoned therapy. To Mr. Schwarz there came the recognition that any hope lay not in the terminal stages, but in *Mental Hygiene* and for this goal he has devoted much of his undiminishing energy for decades. The clinic, hospital unit and finally this Institute were developed largely through Mr. Schwarz's irrepressable optimism and determination.

[*] Director of the Institute for Psychosomatic and Psychiatric Research and Training of the Michael Reese Hospital, Chicago, Ill.

On August 11, 1921, the director of the Jewish Social Service Bureau of Chicago opened discussions with the superintendent of the Mandel Clinic of the Michael Reese Hospital concerning an establishment for mental hygiene services. He envisaged several phases of social service work relating to the preparation of psychotic patients for admission to, or discharge from, the Psychopathic Hospital and visits to them at the State Mental Hospitals. Accordingly, early in 1922, a Mental Hygiene department was initiated in the clinic under the direction of Dr. David Levy who was active from 1922 to 1927. In cooperation with one full-time psychiatric social worker he attended two half-day sessions per week, one for children and one for adults.

Almost at once the clinic deviated from the simple objectives for which it was established. In 1922 the first annual report indicated that case work services were classified into categories of intensive therapy, short term services without full responsibility and steering functions. It soon became apparent that the personnel of the social agencies of the community and of the clinic itself were unable to come to terms regarding relegation of function and responsibility for psychiatric services. Although it seemed at the time that the first year of the psychiatric clinic's existence was a critical period because of this controversy, perusal of volumes of correspondence and stacks of documents relating to the position, function, responsibility, etc. of the psychiatric clinic and the agencies reveals the surprising fact that from 1922 to the present time such conflicts regarding responsibility for psychiatric services remain constant.

I shall not mention the many names of the psychiatrists, psychologists, and psychiatric social workers who have been associated with the clinic during the past quarter century and who are now distinguished teachers, clinicians and investigators. Study of their activities through annual reports indicate that they all suffered through the many vicissitudes that accompany a growing discipline. Troubles within the organization, conflicts with other medical specialties and with more or less cooperating agencies made life interesting albeit a trifle rough.

Before 1925 the now classical psychiatric, psychologic and psychiatric social service team was organized; diagnostic, intaking and agency staff conferences were held regularly and varying goals of therapy were planned for each case. In 1925 undergraduate Smith College students were accepted for training in psychiatric social work and in 1927 an occupational therapy workshop was developed for out-patients. In 1928 after moving to the new Mandel Clinic building on the Michael Reese Hospital campus, although still functioning with inadequate rooms designed primarily for medical or surgical work, the volume of demand for psychiatric services sharply rose and has continued to increase throughout the years. To maintain a high standard of patient care it has become apparent that quality rather than quantity of care must always be our objective and that responsibility for the community's needs can never be accepted or achieved.

In 1933 Mrs. Clara Bassett, under the direction of the National Committee for Mental Hygiene, surveyed our facilities and the community's needs and recommended a staff of full-time psychiatrists. This was accepted but not implemented for several years. Also during this year the University of Chicago's School of Social Service Administration established a field work center at Michael Reese and the Smith College affiliation was terminated. In the subsequent seventeen years our relationship with the University has become increasingly closer in teaching and in research and ever more mutually profitable. Finally in 1936 a department of psychiatry staffed by full-time workers was organized under the direction of Dr. Jacob Kasanin. Several psychiatric residents and assistants were also employed and Dr. Martha MacDonald developed child psychiatry in the clinic and in the Pediatric Hospital to a high level of service. Dr. Samuel J. Beck arrived in 1936 to organize the now flourishing psychology laboratory. In 1939 the first in-patient psychiatric unit with ten beds was opened on an experimental basis for one year but only today, twelve years later, do we relinquish this unit, grown to twenty-two beds and containing a wide diversity of therapeutic and research facilities.

In 1942 World War II decimated the department, leaving Dr. Maxwell Gitelson and Dr. Emmy Sylvester full-time director of the Psychiatric Services and Child Psychiatry respectively alone with a single resident, Dr. David Wheeler, to carry on successfully the prodigious task of keeping the departmental facilities functioning in clinic and hospital. In 1945, at the end of the war, this new Institute entered the planning stage and ground was broken in 1949. In the meantime additional temporary research facilities were acquired, psychiatric services increased and the teaching program for psychiatric residents, psychology externes, psychiatric social service students and psychosomatically interested internists was expanded. In 1949 a new clinic floor was constructed especially for our out-patient psychiatric services, giving us private treatment rooms and the development of many other needed facilities.

Finally today we open our new Institute for Psychosomatic and Psychiatric Research and Training which is well equipped with the most modern patients' rooms, public space, occupational therapy, research laboratories of all types, teaching facilities, etc. The hospital section contains eighty beds divided into four divisions for the care and study of psychosomatic problems and all phases of psychotic disorders of children and adults.

In our development since 1922 there has been constant emphasis on clinical dynamic psychiatry in its broadest sense. Recently we have been able to construct and utilize biochemical, physiological and psychological laboratories which gave to our research and teaching the beginnings of a multi-disciplinary approach. In the new Institute we plan to emphasize that clinical psychiatry as represented by the study of the patient himself is only one small facet of the investigation of human behavior and its disorders. It is our conviction that from the morphological to the social sciences, all disciplines devoted to the study of the functioning of man, part and whole, are concerned in what can be called psychiatry. Perhaps we should state that we are actually dealing with the science of behavior that takes into consideration part and total functions of healthy and sick human beings as they influence and are influenced by interpersonal relations. Therefore, you see on the program today several highly specialized distinguished investigators who come to present summaries of the present state of development in their disciplines as they apply to the behavioral science and predictions as to what their particular fields may contribute in the future. Unfortunately, time and space do not permit us to include all the activities nor all the individuals we would have liked.

It is our hope that a multi-disciplinary group such as is represented here today may contribute, with help from other fields, to a unified theory of human behavior through processes of integrating data and communicating these to each other in common terms without the strains of translation or the creation of a new vocabulary. From contributions of today and many other days to come an integration may be achieved to point the way to hypotheses and procedures which will lead to newer concepts of relationships between the parts and the whole of man as they express themselves in human functions and as they develop and react in response to environmental forces. It is to such a multi-disciplinary approach that this Institute is dedicated in its research, in its teaching and, as far as knowledge is available, in its maintenance of health and the care of the sick.

II

CORTEX AND MIND

By
Percival Bailey*

> Deep, deep, and still deep and
> deeper must we go, if we would
> find out the heart of a man.
> —Herman Melville

In 1665 Niels Steenson[51] (Nicolaus Steno) gave a talk on the brain at the home of Melchisedech Thévenot, a wealthy patron of science in Paris, in the course of which he said: "I am nevertheless very much convinced that they, who seek for solid knowledge, will find nothing satisfactory in all that has been written about the Brain, but it is very certain that it is the principal Organ of the Soul, and the Instrument by which it works very wonderful Effects." Nor do we find any satisfaction today if we try to study the brain only as the organ of the soul which is impalpable and immeasurable. From this point of view we can arrive only at the conclusion of the psychoanalyst that the study of the nervous system adds nothing to our understanding of the behavior of human beings.

Our conclusion becomes quite different, however, if we look at the brain from the standpoint of the theory of evolution which demands that mental operations be derived from ordinary physical principles by progressive steps.[31] From this point of view the nervous system may be considered as a mechanism for the transmission of signals which arise in the peripheral sense organs, are transmitted by the sensory nerves as pulses of electrical potential to the central nervous system, and there are variously in-

* Professor of Neurology and Neurosurgery, University of Illinois Medical School, Director of the Illinois State Psychopathic Institute.

tegrated and then reflected over the motor nerves to result in our behavior.[21]   Their integration in the spinal cord is relatively simple and invariable; that in the cerebral cortex is fluctuant and relatively unpredictable.[41]   The handling of signals in the brain has never been understandable by analogy with such inflexible machines as telephone systems, juke boxes or harpsichords,[35] and this has been a chief stumbling-block to understanding it as a machine.   But, since the invention of the thermionic valve, it has been possible to construct machines that have many of the properties heretofore believed to be peculiar to the brain.   Such machines seek goals, learn, forget, foresee and avoid dilemmas and, in other ways, comport themselves like living beings.

It has been shown that the cerebral cortex, under certain circumstances, acts like a computing machine, such as is used for radar control of anti-aircraft guns, responding to misalignment by giving a neural response calculated to reduce the misalignment, thus correcting its error by the process known as negative feedback.[16]   Such mechanisms have long been known to physiologists and psychologists; only the name "feedback," borrowed from engineering, is new.[48]   It means only the joining of a receptor and an effector in such a way that the receptor cannot only stimulate the effector but also be stimulated by it.   Together with the external world the cerebral cortex forms such a dynamic system which tends to reach a stable equilibrium and improves its stability against disturbance.[2]   Its structure is entirely compatible with such an analogy, because of its vast areas of random neural nets and self-reexciting chains[32] between input and output.

For a long time our ideas concerning the structure of the cerebral cortex were confused by the erroneous hypothesis that it consists of a mosaic of organs.[11]   This was doubtless due to the persistent influence of Franz Joseph Gall.   In accordance with this hypothesis the anatomist's task was to locate and delimit areas of special structure since a difference in structure implies a difference in function.[26]   The physiologist could then investigate the functions of the organs so identified.   This method of approach was clearly stated by Meynert from his study of the striate area and was encouraged by the discovery of the large cells in the precentral gyrus by Betz; the striate area was shown to be concerned with vision and the Betz-cell area with motion of the skeletal muscles. And so the search was on for other areas of specific structure and function. The search resulted in the discovery of two other regions whose structure approached that of the striate area in that they tended to be formed of small cells, so that Economo called them koniocortices,[18] which have been shown to be the regions where the auditory and somesthetic impulses, respectively, arrive at the cortex. The greater part of the cortex, however, was found to have a six-layered structure so similar that students of cytoarchitectonics have been unable to come to any consensus as to its important subdivisions. Nevertheless, elaborate maps have been made and extensively used by physiologists who forgot that, if a difference in structure means a difference in function, the corollary may also be true and areas of essentially identical structure have the same function, insofar as that function depends on the intrinsic structure.[8]

Since the cortex is a communication machine its functioning must also be determined in large part by its extrinsic connections. These connections are now known in considerable detail and they make it clear that the isocortex may best be understood by considering it as one machine for handling signals.[10] The inputs for visual, somesthetic and auditory signals are known, as we have just remarked, and the main output also. We are not surprised that both have relatively fixed mosaic patterns of organization, nor that the structure of the input differs from that of the output. But what of the vast remainder of the isocortex which has a practically uniform structure? It consists, so far as we now know, of myriads of nerve nets,[34] primordially random, capable of being connected together in an infinity of ways under the impact of experience so that its patterns are dynamic and fluctuating. As Hughlings Jackson pointed out long ago,[26] it is necessary that we begin with an unorganized and readily modifiable cortex, otherwise we could not make adjustments to new circumstances. How the definitive connections are made during development we do not know, but Ashby[3] has proven that it is possible for a machine, provided it is furnished with a sufficient number of step-functions. The cortex has a sufficiently vast number,[23] since it is composed of neurones which discharge or else not, in accordance with the well-known all-or-none law, automatically to change its connections until it reaches a successful combination.

The greater part of the cortex, then, composed of neuronal nets arranged somewhat at random at first, completes its structural organization some time after birth and modifies its functional organization constantly by the interaction of new experience with old experience retained in the form of memories. In order for the cortex continually to alter its organization in this way it is necessary that its equilibrium be dynamic, a multitude of parts being free to interact with one another after the manner of feedbacks. There is abundant evidence, since the initial demonstration of Hans Berger, of the dynamic nature of the cortex and Grey Walter[53] has shown that it is possible, by altering the feedback relationships, to cause serious perturbations of its functioning, even epileptic attacks.

However random may be the horizontal organization of the cortex, we must not forget that it has a very definite vertical organization in six layers. The significance of this arrangement is not known but Craik[15] supposed that it might imply a scanning mechanism and this scanning was related by Grey Walter[52] to the alpha rhythm. Pitts and McCulloch[46] have shown how such a mechanism might enable the cortex to recognize universals, such as chord regardless of pitch, or shape regardless of size. This ability is the so-called suprasensuous reason—the power to indicate universals and relate them one to another.

Most of these hypotheses need a great deal of experimental work in support but they already point the way to the understanding of many matters heretofore thought to be outside the realm of scientific investigation, such as curiosity, foresight or free will.

Many years ago Hughlings Jackson[26] maintained that the highest level of nervous activity—the mind—had two aspects—intellect and emotion—and that these activities went on in the cortical areas of generalized structure, then called the associational areas. He maintained further that the greater part of mentation went on in the form of visual images. Certainly visual images play a large role in many forms of thought but a great deal of it goes on in the form of internalized conversation, as George H. Mead[38] has so conclusively demonstrated. This sort of internalized activity, whether visual, auditory or other, is the characteristic activity of large areas of the cerebral cortex and all the evidence which we have at present indicates that it goes on predominantly in the areas of generalized structure, previously known as the associational areas. Now machines have recently been built which behave in a strangely similar manner. A good example is Ashby's homeostat[5] which, by internal self-induced action and interaction, adapts to a disturbance by rearranging its own wiring so as to reach a new state in equilibrium with the new conditions. This is essentially the process of thought. By means of this process tentative solutions are compared with memories of previous solutions, and of their results, and a new combination is reached in relation to the new conditions. This is perhaps the most distinctive property of the human cortex.[23]

During all this process of internal activity the output is blocked; the ultimate result is normally an external activity of the machine directed towards its environment. This external activity has for its purpose to alter or abolish the conditions which disturbed the state of equilibrium in the dynamic system. For this purpose much energy may be necessary, the source, nature and necessity of which are imperfectly understood.[24] The quarter of a kilogram-calory[36] per minute furnished by the oxidation of glucose in the brain is undoubtedly sufficient for the transmission of signals, since communication machines need only small amounts of energy for such activity, but the brain is a living organism and needs other materials for its trophic processes. The greatest students of abnormal psychology have found it necessary to postulate sources of energy for the apparatus of the mind; Janet[30] based a whole system of psychology on the fluctuation and economical administration of this energy and Freud[22] looked forward to the possibility of influencing its amount and distribution by chemical means. If we understand the vague sense in which they used the word "energy" as something necessary for the healthy functioning of the cortical neurones we must agree with them.

Cannon[12] has extensively investigated the mechanisms utilized by the body to mobilize energy. Whenever the external action follows almost immediately upon the disturbance which aroused it, these mechanisms operate smoothly but, when the external action is blocked and unutilized, energy accumulates in the organism and perturbations are produced of which we become aware as emotions. The common man has long recognized that one way out of this situation is to "blow off steam" like a steam-engine, in ways not adapted to the goal of removing the initiating disturbance, such as weeping, ranting and raving, aimless activity, trembling and sweating. It is common parlance to say that these relief activities are caused by the emotions. This ignores the fact that an emotion is itself a derivative phenomenon and causes nothing, being aroused by the disturbance to which it is necessary to adapt. This disturbance is the cause of all the activity which goes on in the dynamic system, as well the internal travail (thought) as the derivative phenomena (emotion) and finally the external activity (behavior).

If we look at the cerebral cortex in this way, as a machine, the apparent conflict between psychogenesis and somatogenesis begins to evaporate. A machine may function badly because it was constructed from inferior materials, because of water in the gasoline, because of rusting from being left out in the weather, because of long hard usage, or merely from overloading. Of course, an inferior machine will break down sooner from overloading but even the best machine has its limits. In the same way a nervous system may function badly because of hereditary or congenital defect, because of improper food supply, because of being soaked in alcohol, because of constant wear from interminable conflict or from a single overwhelming crisis.

It is futile to talk of the effect of the mind on the body. Thought is a name we give to the functioning of our thinking-machine (cortex) just as flight is a name we give to the functioning of flying-machines (airplanes). The plane is worn out *during* flight, but not *by* flight; it is worn out by friction of the air, of the crank-shafts, by buffeting from wind and weather. Our cerebral cortex is worn out also by the buffeting of the environment, both internal and external, which gives rise to thought and, if too severe, causes it to knock or chatter in its functioning which we call the mind.

It follows that there are many ways to remedy the malfunction.

It is not possible to remove a defective part of our cerebral cortex and replace it with a better in any particular machine but we may, by proper genetic procedures, by better maternal care or by prevention of disease during development, see to it that future human machines function better and are built of better materials. And we can see to it that the defective machines are not set to tasks beyond their strength. We can see to it that our human machines are given the proper fuels and lubricants, that they are properly cared for and that damaging intoxicants or poisons are eliminated. They may even function better for certain limited tasks if parts are removed, as by lobotomy, thus removing harmful reverberating chains.[32] We may remove them from environments where heavy tasks are too often set them. We may find them other tasks better fitted to their capacity. By means of drugs we may reduce the sensitivity of certain receptors on which the functioning depends or increase certain resisters which will change the flow of power within the machine.

You may agree with all this and yet say that this does not explain those things which are peculiar to the human machine—purpose, adaptability, foresight. On the crude analogy to an automobile, an airplane, or a telephone exchange—even an automatic one—much will remain obscure and it would be presumptuous to say everything is now understood. Yet machines have been built which follow goals, explore, learn. By analogy with these new machines which learn, correct their errors, break down if their feedbacks are maladjusted, we begin to see more deeply into these formerly mysterious matters and, the deeper we penetrate, the more the fog begins to dissipate and it becomes ever clearer that the concepts which we gather under the term mental are only names given to various aspects of the functioning of the cerebral cortex. It has often been said that we think with our entire body, but it can be readily demonstrated that mental processes go on with negligible disturbance in the absence of all parts of the body below the fifth cervical segment and after most of it is lost above that level except for the brainstem and cortex. The maximal disturbances of the mind result from destruction of the cerebral cortex; the mind is essentially its functioning.

It is even conceivable that it might be possible to build a machine which would have insight, or could be given insight, into its own malfunctioning and take certain measures to correct it. Perhaps this will have to wait until our insight into our own difficulties is less rudimentary. Even so the machine would have to find ways which avoid the necessity to replace a defective part, just as we are unable to replace cortical neurones destroyed by toxins or senile decay, nor can any psychotherapeutist do it for us, and God will not. But the machine can be built to recognize obstacles and avoid them instead of wearing itself out against them. And the mechanic can, by increasing the gain, make it see obstacles which it previously did not recognize. In the same way the psychotherapeutist can aid our human machine to see an obstacle to our functioning which we may or may not be able to avoid. Mere awareness of a difficulty does not, in spite of the assertions of the analysts and others, guarantee its avoidance and the proper functioning of the machine.

The cerebral cortex is, therefore, a machine—a machine for handling signals. That does not mean that it is only a machine, nor is it all of the brain. Hughlings Jackson used the word consciousness as synonymous with mentation but we know from the work of Janet, Freud and others[25] that processes go on while we are asleep or under the influence of an anesthetic which, when we are aware of them, we call thought. Identification of consciousness with the mind leads to much confusion and the resolution of the difficulty is usually purely verbal such, for example, as the substitution of the term extraconscious for subconscious.[13] The distinction of consciousness from the mind leads to its being chased out of the cortex and down through the basal ganglia,[17] the hypothalamus[45] and the midbrain[6] into the bulb.[20]

The soul also has been chased about in the brain. It has been said that the human being is more than a machine because he suffers and is conscious that he suffers. Then a dog must also be more than a machine. Certainly the anti-vivisectionists believe that dogs suffer and are conscious that they suffer; I know no valid reason to believe otherwise. Do they then have souls? And has a patient, whose frontal lobes have been detached and is no longer conscious of suffering, lost his soul? Buddha said he taught suffering and the relief of suffering. The surgeons have found a much more effective remedy than Buddha's eight-fold way. Or than a psychoanalysis which brings repressed conflicts clearly into consciousness and may as well increase as relieve suffering.

Perhaps the relief of suffering is not a valid goal for a physician.[47] Christianity teaches that only through suffering can one know God and save one's soul. Nevertheless, surgeons are industriously constructing stereotaxic instruments which will enable them to strike more shrewdly at the soul in its very inner citadel.[50] But these matters were best left to the theologians and jurists who, I am sure, will soon be obliged to pronounce upon the legitimacy of these destructive interventions on the brain. Whatever we may think of such concepts as mind, personality, soul, there is no doubt whatever that mutilating operations on the brain alter aspects of human behavior which have been long called by these names. And it does not help our understanding to create a pseudoscientific terminology for such concepts and call them the Superego, the Ego and the Id.[7] The Ego is a resultant of the two forces personified as the Superego and the Id, hence not in the same category. Similarly the mind and the body are concepts of different category and cannot be discussed as two similar persons or forces acting on each other. It is impossible to separate thought from matter that thinks.[42] The mind is merely a name which we give to activity of the cerebral cortex. Mental processes are fragments of the complex conduct of the individual;[39] thought is only a detail and a form of human actions.[29] Only in this sense is it permissible to say that mental activity influences the general behavior of the organism since the response of the cortex will depend on the pattern of its activation at the moment of arrival of a train of impulses. Fragments of this activity may fail to be integrated with the rest, because they arise in an abnormal manner from infection or intoxication, and disrupt the personality so seriously as to result in chronic deliria.[14]

In thermionic machines, to which we have likened the cortex, the goals sought are set by the maker—an airplane, for example, in the case of an anti-aircraft gun. In the case of our human machine the goals were set by God, who created man in His own image, by the insertion of goal-setting mechanisms which make us seek food for self-preservation and the female of the species for self-propagation. These goal-setting mechanisms are very complicated, including hormonal chemical factors as well as nervous ones. The nervous factors lie mainly in older parts of the brain nearer the central canal in what we call the brainstem, paleothalamus and allocortex. The activity of these parts of the nervous system is apt to bring us into conflict with other machines seeking similar goals. These then become essential parts of the environmental disturbance which arouses the behavior of any particular organism. The various methods for controlling and utilizing these interpersonal factors constitute a large part of educational and social theory and practice. It is necessary to make the organism seek other intermediate goals—the acquisition of money, the planting of crops—as necessary factors in reaching a final state of equilibrium. One means of doing this has been extensively investigated by Pavlov[44] and his school and is known as conditioning. This process goes on in the cerebral cortex, to be more specific in the isocortex, and is fostered in the home, schools and churches. The insertion of these derivative intermediate goals delays the reaching of a state of equilibrium in the organism, even until a new world after death, as the result of which a permanent state of unrest is produced which is accompanied by various symptoms of malfunction in the machine. These have to be treated, as before indicated, by the physician or the priest.

As civilization becomes more complicated, and attainment of ultimate goals becomes more delayed, the mechanisms within the isocortex, built up largely by social conditioning since on them depends the smooth functioning of society, need strengthening as against the more individualistic mechanisms seeking the ultimate goals immediately and directly. Even such a fundamental social goal as charity (mutual sympathy and aid) needs constant re-enforcement.[9] This is accomplished largely by words. Words, like other symbols, are information giving rise in the afferent nerves to trains of signals on which the functioning of the cortex depends. Once the cortex has been conditioned to respond to a symbol, as it would to the actual situation to which the symbol refers, the latter becomes a potent factor in the dynamic system, either for good or for evil, for peace or for war.[1]

Words which state that the all-powerful Maker of mankind, who can preserve us even after death, approves of the intermediate goals but disapproves of a fundamental one (such as sexual congress), can be used to block the output of our nervous machine with all the attendant disorders resulting from malfunction. Since God made man in His own image, including the goal-seeking mechanisms which the cortex must control, it was found necessary to adopt, from Zoroaster by way of Mani,[40] a lesser god—a demon known as Satan—to account for these persistent urges which gum up the working of the cortical machine. To those who insist on monotheism Satan must be held to be merely another aspect of the Diety and, if we wish to follow the mystics,[43] so also is Man. It does not clarify matters to rename them the Superego, the Id and the Ego.

When looked at from this point of view the mind-body problem evaporates. Not so that of consciousness. We do not know that any machine built by man has ever been aware of its behavior, even though it be theoretically possible.[54] Although we know that consciousness is closely bound to the nervous mechanisms of the brainstem, no analogy exists in man-made machines which gives a hint towards its understanding. This fact should not deter us from our search. Hope is not necessary to enterprise or success to perseverance. At any rate, we gain nothing by thinking in terms of a paradise before which stands a mythological censor with flaming sword to keep Janet's traumatic reminiscences submerged in a subconscious hell. Whether thinking in terms of reverberating neuronal chains will prove more fruitful remains to be seen. Recent formulations sound again very much like the conceptions expressed long ago by Janet[27] in his study of subconscious fixed ideas only stated, this time, not in anthropomorphic theological terms but in the jargon of modern engineering. In some way, by free association, hypnosis or otherwise, we must gain access to harmful engrams so as to remove them by reconditioning, or else destroy them by shock therapy or lobotomy without trying to bring them into consciousness.

Having transformed the mind-body problem into the mind-cortex problem and solved it to our own satisfaction, if to no one else's, we are left with a consciousness-brainstem problem. This is the same old problem from a metaphysical standpoint if, indeed, it be a problem at all. My old teacher—Pierre Janet—used to say that the essential error of the metaphysician was to believe that he had a problem.[28] However that may be, the matter will continue to be discussed.[49] Perhaps we could do no better than to end with a statement made by Paul Flechsig[19] concerning the relationship of brain and soul in an address at his Inauguration as Rector of the University of Leipzig. "So long as medical thought remains scientific, and strives to go beyond the immediate practical necessities, outstanding physicians of all civilized nations endeavor to view the arena where the sentient soul labors and where the thinking mind constructs a picture of the world."

REFERENCES

1. ACKERLY, S.: Prefrontal lobes and social development. *Yale J. Biol. & Med.*, 22:471–82, 1950.

2. ASHBY, W. R.: Adaptiveness and equilibrium. *J. Ment. Sc.*, 86: 478–83, 1940.

3. ———: Dynamics of the cerebral cortex: The behavioural properties of systems in equilibrium. *Am. J. Psychol.*, 59:682–86, 1946.

4. ———: Design for a brain. *Electronic Engineering*, 20:379–383, 1948.

5. ———: The Cerebral Mechanism of Intelligent Action. Chap. VI in *Perspectives in Neuropsychiatry* (D. Richter, Ed.). London, Lewis, 1950, pp. 79–95.

6. BAILEY, P.: *Intracranial Tumors.* Springfield, Thomas, 1933, 475 pp.

7. ———: Alterations of behavior produced in cats by lesions in the brainstem. *J. Nerv. & Ment. Dis.*, 107:336–39, 1948.

8. ———: Considérations sur l'organisation et les fonctions du cortex cérébral. *Rev. Neurol.*, 82:1–20, 1950.

9. BARUK, H.: *Psychiatrie morale, expérimentale individuelle et sociale. Haines et réactions de culpabilité.* 2ème édition. Paris, Presses Univ., 1950, 298 pp.

10. BONIN, G. VON: *Essay on the Cerebral Cortex.* Springfield, Thomas, 1950, 150 pp.

11. BRODMANN, K.: *Vergleichende Lokalisationslehre der Grosshirnrinde.* Leipzig, Barth, 1925, 324 pp.

12. CANNON, W. B.: *Bodily Changes in Pain, Hunger, Fear and Rage.* An account of recent researches into the function of emotional excitement. New York, Appleton, 1929, 404 pp.

13. ——: *The Way of an Investigator.* New York, Norton, 1945, 229 pp.
14. Clerambault, G. de: *Oeuvre psychiatrique.* 2 vols. Presses Univ. de France, 1942.
15. Craik, K. J. W.: *The Nature of Explanation.* Cambridge Univ. Press, 1943, pp. 123.
16. ——: Theory of the human operator in control systems. II. Man as an element in a control system. *Brit. J. Psychol., Gen. Sect.,* 38:142–48, 1948.
17. Dandy, W.: The location of the conscious center in the brain—the corpus striatum. *Bull. Johns Hopkins Hosp.,* 79:34–58, 1946.
18. Economo, C. von: *The Cytoarchitectonics of the Human Cerebral Cortex.* Oxford Univ. Press, 1929, 186 pp.
19. Flechsig, P.: *Gehirn und Seele.* Leipzig, Veit, 1896, 112 pp.
20. Foerster, O.: Uber die Bedeutung und Reichweite des Lokalisationsprinzips im Nervensystems. *Verhandl. d. Deutsch. Gesellsch. f. innere Med.* (*Hirnstamm und Psyche,* p. 208), Munich, Bergmann, pp. 117–211, 1934.
21. Forbes, A.: The interpretation of spinal reflexes in terms of present knowledge of nerve conduction. *Physiol. Rev.,* 2:361–414, 1922.
22. Freud, S.: *An Outline of Psychoanalysis.* New York, Norton, 1949, 127 pp.
23. Herrick, C. J.: *Brains of Rats and Men.* Univ. of Chicago Press, 1926, 382 pp.
24. Himwich, A. E.: *Brain Metabolism and Cerebral Disorders.* Baltimore, Williams & Wilkins, 1951, 451 pp.
25. Holmes O. W.: Mechanism in Thought and Morals. Chap. VIII in *Pages from an Old Volume of Life.* Boston, Houghton Mifflin, 1871.
26. Jackson, J. H.: *Selected Writings.* London, Hodder and Stoughton, 2 vols., 1931–32.
27. Janet, P.: *Les névroses et les idées fixes.* Paris, Alcan, 2 vols., 1898.
28. ——: *La pensée intérieure et ses troubles.* Paris, Chahine, 1926, 451 pp.
29. ——: *L'évolution de la mémoire et de la notion du temps.* Paris, Maloine, 1928, 624 pp.
30. ——: *La force et la faiblesse psychologiques.* Paris, Maloine, 1932, 326 pp.
31. Koehler, W.: *The Place of Value in a World of Facts.* New York, Liveright, 1938, 395 pp.

32. Kubie, L.: Theoretical application to some neurological problems of properties of excitation waves which move in closed circuits. *Brain*, 53:166–77, 1930.

33. Lashley, K. S.: The problem of cerebral organization in vision. *Biol. Symposia*, VII:301–322, 1942.

34. Lorente de No, R.: Facilitation of motoneurones. *Am. J. Physiol.* 113:505–23, 1935.

35. McCulloch, W. S.: Modes of functional organization of the cerebral cortex. *Fed. Proc.*, 6:448–52, 1947.

36. ——: The brain as a computing machine. *Electronic Engineering*, 68:492–97, 1949.

37. ——: Physiological processes underlying psychoneuroses. *Proc. Roy. Acad. Med.; Sect. Psychiatr.*, 42:71–80, 1949.

38. Mead, G. H.: *Mind, Self and Society.* Univ. of Chicago Press, 1934, 401 pp.

39. ——: *The Philosophy of the Act.* Chap. XXI. The process of mind, Univ. of Chicago Press, 1938, pp. 357–442.

40. Melamed, S. M.: *Spinoza and Buddha.* Univ. of Chicago Press, 1933, 391 pp.

41. Meyer, A.: Critical Review of the Data and General Methods and Deductions of Modern Neurology. *Collected Papers, I:* 77–148, 1950.

42. Nersoyan, T.: *A Christian Approach to Communism.* London, Muller, 1943, 103 pp.

43. Nicholson, R. A.: The Mystics of Islam. London, Bell and Sons, 1914, 178 pp.

44. Pavlov, I. P.: *Conditioned Reflexes and Psychiatry.* New York, Intern. Publ., 1928, 199 pp.

45. Penfield, W. G.: The Cerebral Cortex and Consciousness. Baltimore, Williams & Wilkins, *Harvey Lectures*, 32:35–69, 1936–37.

46. Pitts, W.; and McCulloch, W. S.: How we know universals: The perception of auditory and visual forms. *Bull. Math. Biophysics*, 9:127–47, 1943.

47. Prick, J. J. G.: La leucotomie est-elle moralement permise du point de vue de ses suites post-opératoires? *Folia. psych., neurol. et neurochir. Néerlandica.*, 52:391–400, 1949.

48. Rosenblueth, A.; Wiener, N.; and Bigelow, J.: Behavior, purpose and teleology. *Phil. Sc.*, 10:18–24, 1943.

49. Ryle, G.: *The Concept of Mind.* London, Hutchinson, 1949, 334 pp.

50. SPIEGEL, E. A.; WYCIS, H. T.; MARKS, M.; AND LEE, A. J.: A stereotaxic apparatus for operations on the human brain. *Science, 106*:349–50, 1947.
51. STENO, NICOLAUS: *A Dissertation on the Anatomy of the Brain.* Copenhagen, Busck, 1950, 50 pp.
52. WALTER, W. G.: Features in the electrophysiology of mental mechanisms. *Perspectives in Neuropsychiatry.* London, Lewis, 1950, pp. 67–78.
53. ——: The functions of electrical rhythms in the brain. *J. Ment. Sc., 96*:1–31, 1950.
54. WEINBERG, M.: Mechanism in neurosis. *American Scientist, 39:* 74–99, 1951.

III

NEUROPHYSIOLOGY IN RELATION TO BEHAVIOR

By

RALPH W. GERARD[*]

A couple of months ago, at a meeting of the Macy Conference on Cybernetics, Claude Shannon exhibited a rough model of an electric mouse which went through a maze of 25 squares, 5 x 5, and, after exploring it thoroughly, once, then proceeded to run it perfectly. This kind of learning, I am sure, could not be duplicated by the people in this room, certainly not if the maze were made a little larger, which would be no technical problem. Nevertheless, no one believes that that instrument has a mind, and I am sure only the most hard-boiled Cybernetists would say it had a brain. All that was involved was that the circuits were triggered so that the machine left each square the next time round in the same direction that it last left on the first time round. Other machines have been made, as Dr. Bailey has elaborated, that can do a great many other things; but, perhaps in slight disagreement with his views, I would maintain that none of them, even conceptually, as yet can begin to duplicate the neural capacities of the simplest mammalian brain.

Certainly a major objective of this Institute is to study the nuances of human behavior, and so ultimately to get at the neural mechanisms with which they are associated. Like Dr. Bailey, I am sure I can assume that no one in this audience seriously doubts the intimate association of brain and mind. The problem of neurophysiology is that of working out the neural mechanisms of behavior, and with the same objective of ultimately improving

[*] Professor of Physiology, The University of Chicago.

human welfare, so that it is no accident that physiology and psychiatry find their paths often running very much in parallel.

There are some doubts, however. Physiology is universally recognized as a science, and concerned therefore with the predictable and the regular, whereas behavior is notoriously unpredictable and irregular. I am sure most of you have heard that famous Harvard law of animal behavior: Under the most carefully controlled experimental conditions, animals behave as they damned please.

The psychiatrists present recognize very important regularities, however, even in the play of human behavior; and so does the layman. Let us assume that the problem is soluble. The range of behavior that must some day be accounted for in terms of neural mechanisms includes not only the normal but all the variations of consciousness and self-awareness; of learning, remembering and recalling; of ideation and imagination; of emotion, drive and purpose; of the organization of raw sensation into percepts; and, on the motor side, of the performance of coordinated time sequences of movements often individually acquired.

To account for these we have an apparently very meager set of properties with which to work. We have only the attributes of the individual unit and the attributes of the interconnections of those units. One might take some courage from the fact that all of our language is built up from only twenty-six units in various combinations—or, for that matter, that all the material universe is built from a handful of sub-atomic particles in their various interconnections. Still, the problem is enormously difficult.

The units, of course, are the neurons, some ten billion of them, each of which in turn is composed of perhaps a million billion individual molecules and ions. The individual neuron, by virtue of the great number of sub-units that compose it, is able to exhibit a continuous spectrum of change—what in engineering or communication terms is often called analogical behavior—in that the individual neuron's threshold, electrical potential, metabolic rate, and the number and timing of the discharges it makes, is variable.

It is at this level particularly, I think, that the whole chemical story comes in: changes in metabolism induced by changes in the chemical surround and in the composition of the cell. But this is a complete story in itself, that I shall omit. I would express my own faith, however, that in the foreseeable future, a matter of a decade or two, this is the most likely line of advance toward the practical solution, with effective treatment, of the major psychoses, at least of schizophrenia.

The message that is set up by the neuron is discontinuous. It is all or none. It is there or not there. It behaves, as the communication and calculating machine people would say, in a digital fashion. Because of this, and because of the rigid morphology attributed to the nervous system, the picture that had been in existence until fairly recently was the one to which Dr. Bailey has also alluded—the telephone exchange analogy—in which the rigidity of time, space and quantity is terrific. Only one-sized message could go. The times involved were only those for stimulus of the receptor, conduction along a variety of paths, and passage out to the effector, leaving no basis for times of more than a few thousandths of a second. Position was fixed, in that a message getting into one particular fiber went to specific connections and could activate or fail to activate only the pre-connected cells; there was no possibility of flexibility, learning, modification.

We have learned in the intervening time that the rigidity of the nerve fiber and its impulse and the rigidity of the connection, the synapse, are not nearly so great as we had believed. There are considerable freedoms introduced at that level. Still more, we have recognized the error of thinking, as Eddington so well put it, that when we knew one we knew two because one and one make two; we have discovered that we need to know a great deal more about "and." I would say that the burning point of neurophysiological thought and advance today is just in this area of the "and."

This carries us on, then, from the individual unit to the second part of our resources, the interconnections, and their mechanisms and patterns. I should like to speak first about the mechanisms of the interconnections, and then the patterns. Incidentally, at this point also one of the great debates is going on in neurophysiology on the extent to which the nervous system as a whole can be subsumed under the notion of a digital type of instrument, or of an analogical type, or the extent to which each operates.

Concerning the mechanisms, first let me remind you of that tremendously important finding by Berger, that rhythmicity, automaticity, spontaneity of action of the neurons of the nervous system, exists. That has a number of major theoretical consequences, aside from its practical usefulness in the clinic in the EEG machine. It at once gives the possibility of an internal clock; if there is some timed rhythm, then there might be some way of counting the ticks and getting subjective time. More important, if units can be spontaneously active, then it is obviously true that one has a symmetrical possibility of change. They not only can be raised from an inactive state to an active state, which constitutes excitation, but they can also be lowered from an active to an inactive state, which constitutes inhibition. And so, as had been known in fact for some time, inhibition in the central nervous system (and I am using the term physiologically) is just as extensive and important as is excitation. Inhibition is not the absence of positive excitation but the presence of a negative quantity.

Secondly, I would like to emphasize that changes in the state of activity of a given neuron, whether to increase or decrease it, can be brought about by what I might call field effects, quite independently of the impingement of nerve impulses upon that neuron. There are two sorts of field effects which can roughly be called chemical and physical.

On the chemical side, neurons can be thrown into activity or thrown out of activity by a tremendous variety of changes in their environment: changes coming through the blood; changes made possible in the intercellular fluid, without changes in the blood, by alterations in the blood-brain barrier; changes produced by the redistribution of molecules and particularly salt ions between the interior and exterior of individual neurons (and if they get to the outside of some they can affect other neurons); changes due to the actual liberation of specific substances, neuro-hormones and neurohumors, perhaps, from neurons, which, by straight diffusion to neighboring units, can influence their activity. I would remind you of the extreme case of strychnine which fires off neurons to which it is applied, of the discharge and blocking which can be produced by lack of oxygen, altered CO_2, carbohydrate decrease, change in the ratio of calcium and potassium and, of course, of those more subtle chemical alterations produced by the hormones, which are manifested in the behavioral properties of the nervous system. There are certainly important chemical field effects whereby neurons can be altered in their state of activity, independently of the arrival of nerve impulses over nerve fibers and along nerve nets, fixed or flexible.

Even more important, I am satisfied, are the physical fields. There are a number possible, but no reason to invoke most of them. At one time I toyed with the notion of radiation fields, it seemed then that mitogenetic rays might exist, but this now appears sterile. There is no reason to suspect mechanical effects of one neuron on another. But there is a tremendous amount of evidence documenting the importance of electrical fields and their influences.

It is nice to remember, sometimes, that, whereas no organism has a receptor specialized for the detection of electrical changes in the environment, nevertheless the nerve fiber, the entire neurone, is more sensitive to electrical stimuli by far than to any other kind. It is sensitive to such a degree that for practically half a century response of a nerve constituted the most sensitive electric current detecting device available to man. It seems unlikely that there would be this extraordinary sensitivity to electrical currents unless they had some significance to those units. And, of course, they do.

As you know, a neuron never can become active without rather a large electrical change, the action potential. There is quite convincing evidence that the propagation of the nerve impulse itself depends on the existence of these electrical eddy currents between one region and another. Changing the electrical field in which a neuron finds itself—either sharply, which gives it an acute stimulus as in electroshock; or even gradually, which alters the steady potential field of the nervous system—produces marked changes in neural activity. One can start or stop spontaneous rhythms in the brain by polarization with extremely feeble currents, ones of the order of those which actually appear in the nervous system spontaneously. Moreover, there is good reason to believe that large numbers of neurons can enter into synchronous activity, which alone makes possible the recording of such a thing as an

EEG, or they even can become active in sequential activity, as in propagating waves over the cerebrum; and all this modifiable by changes in the internal or applied electric fields to which they are exposed. I would emphasize the importance of field effects as part of the important mechanisms in integrating the neurons in their interactions.

The third point as regards the mechanism of interactions is, of course, the flow of impulses along connections and acting at synaptic junctions. Here also is a region that is quite active in neurophysiology and pharmacology and biochemistry, the exact mechanism whereby an impulse arriving at an axon terminal successfully excites the neuron across the synapse, the post-synaptic element. I think most neurophysiologists are strongly convinced that this mechanism is also electrical in the central nervous system. In some of the peripheral junctions it is very probably a chemical mechanism. Be that as it may, here also there are extremely few variables with which to manipulate. There is every reason to believe that all nerve impulses are qualitatively alike. There are not different kinds of nerve impulses and, as far as I know, there is no good evidence that this is not the case for the synapse. There is no different kind of a synapse for an inhibitory and an excitatory impulse, any more than the impulse going along the nerve fiber is different in the two cases.

That leaves us, then, with these possible parameters to play with: The number of synapses activated by a particular nerve fiber; the effectiveness of any given synapse, whether it alone produces a big enough change to excite or only when active in conjunction with other synaptic endings; the spatial distribution of these endings on the cell body or dendrites; and the time pattern of the impulses that arrive at the synaptic endings. This is not a great deal, but even this much has made possible the understanding of much neural functioning. We recognize perfectly valid and clear-cut mechanisms with just these variables involving one kind of ending, which account for excitation, summation, facilitation and inhibition. The effect of different temporal patterns of impulses can be shown, in many instances, by stimulating an afferent nerve with identical shocks at different frequencies. One produces at one frequency a positive reflex and at a different frequency a negative one. Inspiration or expiration, swallowing or no swallowing can be induced just by changing the pattern of timing of the input impulses. That can now be interpreted. Even some understanding of conditioning can be obtained at this synaptic level.

Most of the behavioral properties upon which we wish enlightenment, however, must be understood, if at all, in terms of the patterns of interaction rather than of the mechanisms of interaction. There are three things I would like to bring out about the patterns.

First, and indubitably of great importance, are the nerve nets, especially with the possibility, mentioned several times, of reverberating circuits. These are chains of neurones, or perhaps three-dimensional nets, which close upon themselves; so that an impulse entering the assembly can travel through it, find itself back at the beginning, and so continue to go round and round, as well as being able to leave along axone branches to various effectors and to maintain responses. This, you see, at once takes away the time rigidity. Things can go on happening in the nervous system, theoretically, indefinitely after a stimulus, because this trapped wave can continue to go round and round; as, indeed, a trapped wave in the mantle of a jellyfish was once made to circulate for ten days and travel six hundred odd miles—until the investigator got tired. Besides giving freedom in time, such circuits exemplify the very essence of the notion of closure and Gestalt; they close on themselves to produce "wholes." They offer the possibility of explaining, as Dr. Bailey has already elaborated, the feed-back story, behavior directed toward a changing goal. Servomechanisms behave the same way, the homing torpedo or anti-aircraft shell; and, looked at objectively, such mechanisms exhibit purpose. We have here, then, potentially an explanation of purpose. Such mechanisms have also been invoked to explain memory, particularly recent dynamic memory, such as I am now using in remembering what I am going to say for the next few minutes (by tomorrow I would not have it in mind). Such transient memories could be well accounted for in terms of reverberating circuits that keep going for a time. They are not efficient mechanisms if they do exist, but they have rich possibilities of explaining behavior.

I hesitate to sound a slightly negative note regarding this thesis at this time, but I am personally a bit afraid that the reverberating circuit notion has been overplayed. For one thing, although gross circuits, such as the feedback ones between cortex and thalamus, cerebellum and basal ganglia, spinal cord and muscle, are certainly there, to my knowledge no one has yet demonstrated the actual existence of a reverberating circuit on anything like the micro or semi-micro level at which we often invoke it. For another thing, and directly concerning memory, some experiments being done by Mr. Ransmeier in my laboratory are giving negative results. If even recent memory depends upon such circuits, the question has always arisen, how does memory continue after sleep or coma? The answer has been that the circuits have not been sufficiently disturbed in these conditions.

We have taken advantage of the hibernating ability of rodents, and have cooled hamsters to temperatures of 4°C. At this level they are completely unable to give any reflexes, every measurable activity of the nervous system is gone, including any kind of spontaneous or evoked electrical responses, and respiration is so nearly stopped that one sometimes must look at the exposed heart to tell whether an animal is alive. Nevertheless, such hamsters, having been taught a few days before to run a maze, when warmed up after several hours of refrigeration and put back to their problems, perform as well as before the cooling. Their recent memory has in no way been impaired by stopping all possible active circuits in the brain. One can do the same thing in reverse by intense electroshock, which would also effectively break up any such dynamic circuits; again hamsters so shocked show no loss of recent memory although shocks can produce deterioration of learning.

The other mechanism of interaction, the field, I have already alluded to. This also gives us many possible types of explanation which we did not have previously. It gives us at once, and we greet it with a sigh of relief, freedom from the particular neural unit. For when a field of activity, say a pattern of electrical potential, is set up in an area of the brain, it does not matter whether one particular cell or its immediate neighbor or even a cell some little distance away is exactly at the peak of the potential map. It is the topography as a whole that counts. Any one of a number of units might be involved with any one of a considerable number of other units, and there results that very necessary freedom from the telephone line type of connection. With such field mechanisms it is not difficult to explain conditioning. Koehler has used some of these findings to account for optical illusions in man. The formation of dynamic motor patterns and the fact that abberent muscles, put into effective but abnormal connection with the spinal cord, pick up and respond in the normal manner to these patterns—all these things can be accounted for best in terms of dynamic fields.

One last type of pattern I must mention very sketchily. When one considers the myriad neurons, of units, which are probably involved in any kind of behavioral activity, perhaps the argument between digital and analogical functioning loses some of its force. Just as the billions of molecules and ions in the neuron give it a continuous range of performance, so also, if thousands or millions of neurons are involved in a particular activity, they might collectively behave as an analogical continuum. In any event, statistical approaches to behavior, making use of such concepts, look extremely interesting.

With appropriate assumptions about a statistical variation in the properties of neurons, and accepting, as has been demonstrated experimentally on the single nerve fiber, that the threshold of each unit can fluctuate following a probability curve (mostly the threshold is at some level, but it may at any moment be a little above or a little below, more rarely far above or far below), with such probablistic and statistical considerations it is possible to see how the nervous system, and perhaps even ultimately a man-made machine, could produce the novel. It could form new and indeterminate patterns and so exhibit creativity and imagination and get new ideas about the world.

It is still a long way from our present stage of neurophysiology to an adequate explanation of human behavior or, for that matter, of even simple animal behavior. However, it is clear now, I think, that we are on the way, and that the kind of knowledge and thinking going on in this field is potentially and foreseeably able, even without any major new kinds of discoveries (which surely will occur), to account for human behavior.

I will close with a quotation, not from any of the distinguished fathers of psychiatry or neurology or physiology, but only from myself. I read this because it was written almost twenty years ago and, I think, it is still essentially valid:

"There are rather striking similarities between the action of an orchestra and that of a brain. In each are many individual units, players or neurons, able to produce a spontaneous rhythm. The units are gathered into groups, not all alike qualitatively, and those within one group, say the first violins, are synchronized by some form of distance action. Dominance occurs within groups and, still more, a leader controls and integrates the activity of the entire ensemble. Even the influence of past events on current activity can be seen in both, in written music or mnemonic traces. The violinists and bassos, each scraping away with his kind, modulating their rhythms to the line of the notes and the baton of the leader, spin out a magnificent pattern of harmony that we call a Beethoven symphony. Similarly, the myriad nerve cells of the brain, as they beat their single rhythms and form and reform their groups and hierarchies, play that greatest harmony of all nature—the totality of animal behavior."

IV

HOMEOSTASIS, BEHAVIORAL ADJUSTMENT AND ThE CONCEPT OF HEALTH AND DISEASE

By

GEORGE L. ENGEL*

This symposium is devoted to the contributions of the con-temporary sciences to mid-century psychiatry. I would like to deviate somewhat from these objectives and to consider instead a unitary concept of health and disease, which focuses more on the contributions of biology and psychology to medicine and on the growth of our understanding of man in process with environ-ment, to paraphrase the transactional view of Bentley.[2] The unitary concept has been perhaps most succinctly stated by Ro-mano,[18] who views health and disease as "phases of life, dependent at any time on the balance maintained by devices, genically and experientially determined, intent on fulfilling needs and on adapt-ing to and mastering stresses as they may arise from within the organism or from without." Health represents the phase of suc-cessful adjustment, disease the phase of failure. Such a concept is by no means new, having been expressed almost a century ago by Claude Bernard,[3] but it has been only very slowly and incom-pletely incorporated into medical teaching and thinking.

Actually the development of a unitary concept of health and disease had to await two important reorientations of man's con-cept of man. Both represented major departures from the pre-vailing ideas of the culture of the times and as such were pro-foundly disturbing and strongly resisted. The first was the growth of a science of biology which recognized the fundamental

---

* Associate Professor of Psychiatry and of Medicine, University of Rochester School of Medicine and Dentistry, Rochester, New York.

sameness of all forms of life and developed the appropriate methodology to study it. The two most important figures responsible for this development were Charles Darwin (1809–1882), and Claude Bernard (1813–1878). Bernard in truth deserves the title of "The Father of Modern Medicine," for he was not only the first to enunciate clearly the dictum that health and disease represent phases of life processes, but he also evolved experimental techniques to demonstrate the validity of this idea.

The second was the development of psychoanalysis, which as a technique and a conceptual framework, has made possible the systematic examination and understanding of human behavior as part of the total adaptation of the organism.

The flowering of 19th century biology and the contributions to it of chemistry and physics greatly stimulated medicine, especially in its practical applications, but significantly even today the currently held concepts of disease tend to exclude from consideration behavior and mental processes. Remnants of demonologic concepts, mechanistic concepts, single cause ideas, and mind-body dichotomy all are reflections of the fact that medical men still are reluctant to consider man's behavior in its broadest sense as a proper subject for scientific study. But without an understanding of behavior and without a scientific psychology, Bernard's advanced views can have application only in a limited sense and chiefly to the infrahuman species. It remained for Sigmund Freud[11] (1856–1939) to provide the concepts and methodology which now allow for the development of a unitary concept of disease. Proof of the influence of dynamic psychology in this development is to be found in the fact that even though psychiatry is the youngest of the medical sciences, the major impetus toward a broadening and unification of the concepts of heath and disease has come in the past decade from psychiatrists and psychologically oriented physicians (Alexander,[1] Dunbar,[10] Halliday,[13], Menninger,[17] Romano,[18] Seguin,[19] to mention only some). Traditional medicine as a whole has tended to resist this growth and to adhere to old and narrow concepts of byegone eras, concepts which exclude from consideration the perplexing and often disturbing implications of man's behavior.

It therefore seems timely to re-examine now some of the background for the dynamic concept of health and disease and to integrate this with modern medical knowledge. In this essay we shall first note some of the specific contributions of Bernard, Darwin and Freud, who lay the groundwork for this concept. We shall then summarize the biological background and the evolutionary aspects in an attempt to delineate the common properties of living organisms and the phylogenetic heritage of man as a living creature. From this point we will consider briefly the transition from the biological to the psychological both in terms of phylogenesis and in terms of the total behavior of man and the higher organisms. This will then provide the necessary background for the elaboration of the unitary concept of health and disease.

CLAUDE BERNARD (1813–1878)

The foundation for the modern concept of disease was layed by Claude Bernard with his brilliantly inspired idea of "le milieu interieur," the internal environment. Bernard emphasized that the conditions necessary for life are found neither in the organism nor in the outer environment, but in both at once. While the outer environment is common to living and to inorganic bodies, the inner environment created by an organism is special to each living being and the capacity to maintain a relative constancy of this internal environment is the condition of life. He considered sickness and death to be "merely a dislocation or disturbance of the mechanism which regulates the contact of vital stimulants with organic units" (1865). While Bernard[4] acknowledged that the understanding of living organisms rests securely upon the physico-chemical sciences, he was aware that biology is more than applied physical science. To quote: "Admitting that vital phenomena rest upon physico-chemical activities, which is the truth, the essence of the problem is not thereby cleared up; for it is no chance encounter of physico-chemical phenomena which constructs each being according to a pre-existing plan, and produces the admirable subordination and the harmonious concert of organic activity.

"Vital phenomena possess indeed their rigorously determined physico-chemical conditions, but at the same time, they subordinate themselves and succeed one another in a pattern and according to a law which pre-exists; they repeat themselves with order, regularity, constancy, and they harmonize in such a manner as to bring about the organization and growth of the individual, animal or plant" (1878).

These views emphasize both the internal and external environments and thereby bring into focus the necessity for considering the spontaneous activities of the organism itself. This is of great importance to the later development of Freud's concept of instincts. To quote further:

"Considered in the general cosmic environment, the functions of man and of the higher animals seem to us, indeed, free and independent of the physico-chemical conditions of the environment, because its actual stimuli are found in an inner organic, liquid environment. . . .

"Living machines are therefore created and constructed in such a way that, in perfecting themselves, they become freer and freer in the general cosmic environment. But the most absolute determinism still obtains, nonetheless, in the inner environment which is separated more and more from the outer cosmic environment, by reason of the same organic development. A living machine keeps up its movement because the inner mechanism of the organism, by acts and forces ceaselessly renewed, repairs the losses involved in the exercise of its functions" (1865).

"A living body, especially in the higher animals, never falls into chemico-physical indifference to the outer environment; it has ceaseless motions, an organic evolution apparently spontaneous and constant; and though this evolution requires outer circumstances for its manifestation, it is nevertheless independent in its advance and modality. As proof of this, we see living beings born, develop, fall ill and die, without the conditions of the external world changing for the observer" (1865).

Thus Bernard's approach to biology is a forerunner of the modern transactional approach of Dewey and Bentley. He saw the organism in action not as something radically set against the environment, but as an integral constituent of a total environment. By defining the conditions of the internal and the external environments, he laid the groundwork for an understanding of the dynamic properties of each and for the types of process to be observed between them. But most important of all, he designed the experimental approach which permitted the scientific examination of these views.

CHARLES DARWIN (1809–1882)

Medicine rarely acknowledges, indeed, hardly seems aware of its indebtedness to Charles Darwin. By establishing the evidence for a developmental continuity between all forms of life he provided the basis for the rational consideration of man as representative of living organisms, a fundamental requirement for physiology and experimental medicine. He greatly stimulated interest in the interrelations between living organisms and their environment, and through the idea of natural selection focused attention on the problems of adaptation as a fundamental area for biological investigation. This was a natural counterpart to Bernard's work.

Gaylord Simpson,[21] in his Terry Lectures of 1948, summarizes the essence of evolutionary theory after almost a hundred years:

"Examined in more detail, the history of life turns out to be an odd and intricate mixture of the oriented and the random. Continuing and clearly oriented trends of evolutionary changes are very common, but when carefully studied without gross oversimplification, they give no appearance of rigid control forcing them in only one direction. They also lack evidence of any vital inner force or momentum that carries them forward regardless of the functional adaptation to way of life or of any random change. The evidence all concurs in suggesting that the orienting force in evolution is neither internal nor external to the organism involved but is in that interplay of both internal and external factors which produces adaptations to way of life and to environment." Claude Bernard's essentially transactional views find support from another quarter.

As a logical outcome of this earlier work on the theory of the evolution Darwin[9] examined more minutely certain details of behavior and published his findings in a book entitled, *Expression of the Emotions in Man and Animals* (1872). Less well known than his works on evolution, this work is important because it represents one of the earliest efforts to examine scientifically behavior in terms of adaptation. Here Darwin considers the expression of emotions in terms of their adaptive functions and at least hints at the idea of maladaptive persistence of originally useful behavior. In brief, he traces some of the observable phenomena of emotional expressions to parts or remnants of movements or activities which functioned in the service of self-preservation in the phylogenetic past or in the infancy of the organism. The expressions of fear and anger, for example, he traced to preparations for flight or struggle. Walter Cannon[6] many years later provided the physiologic evidence to substantiate this hypothesis. Other parts of expression he identifies as means of nonverbal communication, which again form part of the systems of attraction (sexual and social) and defence. "The movements of expression in the face and body, whatever their origins may have been, are in themselves of much importance for our welfare. They serve as the first means of communication between the mother and her infant." The significance of this last observation is only now being appreciated.

Darwin thus performed the monumental task of undermining man's concept of himself as a divinely endowed being apart from other living creatures. By emphasizing the adaptive aspects of the evolutionary process, even though at times in a naive and oversimplified fashion, he opened the way for the consideration of living organisms in process with the environment. It was entirely logical that he soon recognized behavior as part of this adaptive process and devoted study to it. Evolutionary theory provided the much needed link between all the fields of human science, physical, biological, psychological and social.

SIGMUND FREUD (1856–1939)

Freud was obviously influenced by the revolutionary concepts of Bernard and Darwin, although he does not directly acknowledge this. The setting of his early scientific training was one which had been tremendously stimulated by the new biology and evolution. But Freud's interest in the mental processes of sick and healthy people soon led him to the field of psychology and to the early recognition that psychological processes are but one aspect of the function of the higher organisms. Shunning the influence and hostility of the organicists he dared to apply psychological techniques to the study of behavior and to defend their scientific validity as but another approach to the same problems of biology being studied by the chemists, physiologists, pathologists and others.

It is unnecessary—and impossible—to summarize for this audience the contributions to medical thought of Freud and his followers. I wish only to list in a very condensed form certain basic concepts which have application to the subject at hand, namely, the concept of disease: (1) the concept of instincts with their internally and somatically derived energy sources, the same internal forces to which Bernard had reference; (2) the concept of a stable equilibrium, that the organism attempts to satisfy its innate needs, instinctually determined, avoid painful excitation or tension, and maintain an optimum level of excitation and a more or less stable equilibrium (here Freud acknowledges the influence of Fechner, but does not refer to either Bernard or Darwin); (3) the concept of conflict, that various needs within the organism as well as various demands of the external environment upon the organism may be mutually contradictory and hence conflictful; (4) the elucidation of the topography and economics of the psychic apparatus and the proof of the existence of unconscious mental processes; (5) the concept of a danger signal, anxiety, warning of the threat of excess excitation arising from inside or outside the organism and threatening its safety; (6) the concept of defence (more properly adaptation), that is, of the capacity of the psychic apparatus to initiate both psychic and physiologic processes intended simultaneously to avert dangers and assure satisfaction of instinctual needs; (7) the elucidation of the genetics of development, pointing the way to how genic (referring specifically to that which is transmitted through the genes), and experiential factors may determine from conception to death what needs seek expression and through what channels, and what adaptive devices are available and can develop in order to insure the satisfaction of the needs and the avoidance of damage or destruction at each period of development; inherent here is the idea of periods of critical vulnerability, meaning that the organism is more vulnerable to certain stresses at certain periods of development; (8) the principles of inertia and economy which imply that the organism tends to use the successful adaptive devices of bygone periods to meet new stresses even when inappropriate to the current situation; and finally (9) the concept of trauma, the nature of the forces or influences which can seriously disturb the organism's development so that it is thereafter difficult or impossible for the organism to develop beyond a certain stage, to master successfully a similar stress in the future or to meet a new stress. Freud derived these concepts from almost five decades of study of emotionally disturbed and mentally sick people, but as now becomes increasingly evident, these principles contribute a sound basis for a concept of disease in the broadest sense.

THE BIOLOGICAL BACKGROUND

We are now ready to summarize the basic biologic concepts that bear on our understanding of man in process with his environment. To do so it is instructive to begin with the most simple living organism and examine what properties are common to all animals, from amoeba to man:

(1) All organisms manifest spontaneous activity, which is apparent in growth, development and various physiologic processes. The primary energy sources are internal. The limits of these activities for the species are primarily genically determined; the character of the growth, the intra-cellular enzyme composition, the development, and the movement of an amoeba as well as of a man are circumscribed by the original genic constitution. The internal energy sources are probably finite, each organism having a life cycle, a period of rapid growth and development, a relatively stable period, and a period of decline.

(2) All organisms have a limiting surface membrane the intactness of which is essential for the integrity of "le milieu interieur." Disruption of this barrier between internal and external environment is incompatible with life. This membrane functions in a number of specific ways. It is sensitive to many modalities of change in the physical environment. It keeps out that which is noxious (within limits) and permits a continuous exchange of

substances between the two environments, assuring the continuation of and replenishment of the internal energy sources determining life activity and the operation of "self-regulation" to restore balance. These are all requirements for the steady state achieved by the "open" living system in contrast to the "closed" physical system, as outlined by Bertalanffy.[5]

(3) All organisms have the capacity, within limits, to adapt to environmental forces which are damaging to them and thereby minimize or escape injury, and to obtain from the environment what they need for survival, growth, and development. This is genically (as well as phylogenetically) circumscribed and experientially modified. The enzymic constitution, the physico-chemical composition, and the morphology determine as well as limit the capacity of the organism to deal with an environmental process, and also help to circumscribe what might constitute a stressful process. To paraphrase H. S. Jennings,[15] a cornered amoeba cannot escape by flying. We cannot enumerate all the types of adaptive devices found even among unicellular organisms, but a few basic categories might be cited. The organism may accomplish an internal metabolic rearrangement or develop an adaptive enzyme so that a noxious substance becomes harmless or even useful. The antigen-antibody reaction is one example. The organism may utilize motility, moving away from a harmful agent, or toward it if it has special organs of attack, or it may move toward a useful or assimilable object. The organism may have the capacity to retain and ingest or eject a material already ingested. The organism may insulate itself against an unfavorable environment by changing the character of its membrane (i.e., spore or cyst formation). As we will later develop, these constitute the biologic anlage of corresponding psychologic processes in higher organisms. The energy transformations for these processes originate from the internal organization of the organism itself.*

---

* H. S. Jennings, in a classic book, *The Behavior of Lower Organisms* (1906), made very penetrating observations on the essentially regulatory nature of the behavior of the lower organisms under various conditions, indicating the essential unity of such processes in all living beings. By behavior he meant chiefly the ob-

Footnote continued on page 42

Footnote, continued

served movements. This work should be carefully studied by all students of behavior. For the interested reader I quote some of his conclusions:

"The activity of organisms we found to be spontaneous, in the sense that it is due to internal energy, which may be set in operation and even changed in its action without present external stimuli. In reactions this energy is merely released by present external stimuli. What form the activity shall take is limited by the action system, and within these limits is determined by the physiological state of the organism. Physiological states depend on many factors. The two primary classes of states depend on whether the internal life processes are proceeding uninterruptedly in the usual way. Interference with these processes produces a physiological state of a certain character ("negative"), while release from interference or assistance to those processes produces a different state ("positive"). Any change, external or internal, may modify the physiological state, and hence the behavior.

"The effects of external agents depend largely on their relation to the normal course of the life processes—whether aiding or interfering, or neither. A primary fact is that interference with the life processes produces progressive changes in physiological states, inducing repeated changes in behavior. This is in itself regulatory, tending to relieve the interference, whether due to internal or external causes; it is a process of finding a reaction fitted to produce a more favorable condition. When through such changes a fitting reaction is found, the changes in physiological state and hence of behavior cease, since there is no further cause for change. In the same way a fitting reaction to a beneficial change, or one releasing from interference, may be found. This fitting reaction then tends to be preserved, by the law of the resolution of physiological states, in accordance with which the physiological state inducing this reaction is reached more readily after repetition. Thus the production of varied movements by stimulation is the progressive factor in behavior, while the law of the resolution of physiological states is the conservative factor, tending to retain fitting reactions once attained.

"Through the law of the resolution of physiological states behavior tends to pass from the pure 'trial' condition to a more defined state. The operation of this law tends to produce reactions precisely localized, with reference to the position of the stimulating agent; increased appropriate reaction to the first weak effects of injurious or beneficial stimuli; and appropriate reactions to representative stimuli, according as they are followed by injurious or beneficial stimuli."

By representative stimuli Jennings refers to changes that in themselves neither favor nor interfere with the normal life activities, but which do lead to such favor or interference. For example, certain colorless infusoria react to light in such a way as to gather at the lightest side of the vessel. There is no evidence that the light itself is beneficial to them, but their reaction does aid them in obtaining food, since their prey gathers on the lightest side of the vessel. The sea urchin tends to remain in dark places, and light is apparently injurious to it. Yet it responds to a sudden shadow falling upon it by pointing its spines in the direction from which the shadow comes. This action is defensive, serving to protect it from enemies that in approaching may have cast the shadow. The reaction is produced by the shadow, but it refers, in its biological value, to something behind the shadow. In other words, this change has the function of a sign.

(4) All living organisms have the capacity to reproduce and thereby to continue the species. Implicit in this fact is that we may also expect to find behavior which is not self-regulatory but species- or group-regulatory. Such individual behavior also has internal sources and external stimuli and is of profound importance in determining inter-animal relationships. Even among unicellular organisms Jennings observed intricate and complex pairing behavior preparatory to a sexual union in which the intracellular contents are halved and shared, to be followed by extensive reproduction by fission. Significantly, this pairing and conjugation do not take place among the offspring by fission from a common parent or among young or aged organisms. This represents the earliest manifestation of social behavior and bears upon the unity of the manifestations of life in higher and lower organisms.

We are not in position at this time to discuss the intricate problem of the energetics of these processes. For one approach the reader is referred to the paper by Bertalanffy. With him we adhere to the strict determinism of Bernard and Freud and hold that the energy sources are physico-chemical in nature. Bertalanffy compares the "open" system of the living organism with the "closed" physical systems. In the "closed" systems no material enters or leaves, reversibility is in most cases practicable, and an equilibrium-state in which entropy is at a maximum must ultimately be attained. In the "open" biological system, there is a continuous flow of components from without, their flow and ratio are maintained constant, irreversibility appears in great degree, growth is characteristic, a steady-state characterized by minimum entropy-production may be approached, and, finally, when disturbance occurs, "self-regulation" operates to restore balance. To the forces concerned in this tendency of the organism to maintain itself during an organized development and life cycle and to continue the species we would apply Freud's word, *triebe*, or as it has been rendered in English, *instincts*. Hereafter, in using the term instincts or instinctual drives we refer to the primary intrinsic forces underlying the basic biological properties which we have just outlined.

EVOLUTIONARY ASPECTS

Having noted some of the basic biologic functions common to all living organisms it is well now to note briefly the changes wrought through evolutionary progress. The basic instincts do not change and may be considered among the properties common to all living organisms.

Evolution provides a record of the successful and unsuccessful efforts at development of organismic organization to adapt to a changing cosmic environment. The changes that we note express different ways and means of achieving the same end. How instinctual activity is expressed is determined by the particular stage of evolutionary development achieved by the organism, and it is only in the higher organisms, notably man, that we see the representation of the instinctual forces in psychological forms. The spectrum from the purely biological to the psychological can be established by tracing development from the unicellular organism, which contains all its functions within the single cell, to complex man. I shall now attempt to summarize these changes:

(1) As already mentioned the unicellular organism incorporates all functions within the one structural unit, although even some of these animals already show considerable specialization of structure and function within the cell. It has already been pointed out that the basic modes of behavior concerned in survival and reproduction and in the higher organisms have their anlage in the unicellular organisms. The higher organisms, however, manifest these activities at more complex biologic and psychologic levels. Of great importance to our thesis is the discovery by Jennings of the beginnings of social behavior as part of the activity preparatory to sexual union even among unicellular organisms.* It affords evidence that one important impetus for inter-organism relations arises from the basic biologic needs concerned with sexual union and procreation.

(2) Multicellular organisms may be thought to evolve from unicellular organisms through an intermediary stage of colony forma-

---

* Jennings uses social behavior to refer to "the behavior and reactions of individuals with relations to other individuals as such; reactions to individuals as individuals, either singly or in combination, not merely reactions to physical forces or to masses present in the environment."

tion. The development of multicellular organisms requires specialization of function in cells and organs, the development of systems of internal communication and coordination, and systems of external and internal perception. Coordination in the multicellular and multi-organ animal is achieved through the neuro-humoral-system. To trace the development of this system is quite beyond the scope of this paper. Let it suffice to point out certain pertinent steps in the development of the nervous system as it bears on the function of a mental apparatus. With the development of a nervous system a delay is interposed between stimulus and response. Beginning with relatively fixed and circumscribed responses, the progressive development of the central nervous system allows for increased variety and complexity of response, multiple choice, discrimination, retention and utilization of past experience, and in man, abstraction, language, use of symbols, etc., with consequent great economy of function. It is from these developments that the psychic apparatus evolves, but we must not lose sight of its primary biological derivation. The psychological adaptive devices stem directly from biologic anlage. Awareness of self and of one's behavior as an individual among individuals comes with the development of the psychic apparatus, but, as Jennings points out, action and process long precede in evolution such awareness. Gaylord Simpson calls attention to the transition from organic to social evolution in this process:

"It is part of this unique status that in man a new form of evolution begins, overlying and largely dominating the old organic evolution which nevertheless also continues in him. This new form of evolution works in the social structure, as the old evolution does in the breeding population structure, and it depends on learning, the inheritance of knowledge, as the old does on physical inheritance. Its possibility arises from man's intelligence and associated flexibility of response. His reactions depend far less than other organisms on physically inherited factors, far more on learning and on perception of immediate and new situations."

(3) In the service of continuation of the species three important developments occur during evolution. First, the reproductive potential is concentrated in the germ plasm, which alone retains

the capacity to reproduce the whole organism, while the other cells can only reproduce themselves, or at most experience limited metamorphosis.

Second, two sexes are differentiated, although the original basic bisexuality is never lost. The survival value gained from new gene combinations is self-evident. Equally important is the fact that this establishes the necessity for inter-animal relationships to continue the species for in order to mate the male and female must come together in some sort of social relationship. It also leads to differentiation of function between the sexes and the development of specific sexual organs.

The third evolutionary change has to do with the forms of reproduction and the status of the young. The over-all direction of this change can be summarized by saying that there is a wider and wider developmental span between the young and the adult forms. (The insects are a special exception, which need not concern us here.) Two important consequences stem from this, as exemplified in man and the higher animals. First, the young have much greater possibility of experiential and environmental influence as compared to the fixed genically determined patterns of lower organisms. As a result they have not only a greater possibility of flexibility in development but also a greater vulnerability to injury before full development is achieved. The second consequence is a social one, namely, that if the species is to survive the young must be cared for, thus adding a new component to inter-animal relations. Arising from this prolonged dependency of the young we can see the genesis of family and other more complex social units which distinguish the higher organisms, and especially man.

Thus beginning with internally derived instinctual forces having to do with the growth, development, and survival of the individual and of the species, we see the evolution from the single cell to the multicell organism, with subordination of the parts to the whole, and from the relatively isolated to the highly social organism, with the subordination of the organism to the group. There is a continuity between the biologic, psychologic and social evolution.

INSTINCTS: FROM THE BIOLOGICAL TO THE
PSYCHOLOGICAL

We have attempted to point out the consistency of the instinctual sources of energy throughout living organisms and to develop the psychological in continuity with the biological. Some elaboration of this as it applies to man and the higher organisms is in order before we go on to apply this to the unitary concept of health and disease.

We might begin by examining the levels of representation of an imperative need like that for oxygen, necessary for the survival of most organisms. The deficiency of oxygen is perceived by the organism (not consciously at first) and a variety of internal physiological regulatory activities are initiated to compensate for the low oxygen tension and to conserve the supply for the most needed areas. But in addition behavior is initiated in respect to the outer environment, such as efforts to escape or obtain help; or if the deficiency is recognized, recourse may be had to a gas mask or a ventilation device. Indeed in man the danger from oxygen lack eventually contributed to the discovery of oxygen, scientific investigation of respiration, the invention of ventilation systems, and a host of complex social derivatives of the originally biological need and danger. The need is expressed and the adaptations achieved through a broad spectrum of the biological, psychological, and social.

Or we might trace the eventual psychological representation of the biological fact that the materials in the external world which are essential for the growth and survival of the organism must be broken into their elemental components before they can be utilized. The large must be broken into the small in successive stages. It may begin with teeth or claws or a prehensile hand and it is completed by enzymes. Man also enlists tools, machines, fire and chemicals for this purpose. The process may be seen successively at the levels of perception, seizing, handling, ingestion or digestion. Activity is necessary to achieve this, and the activity originates from the stimulus of the instinctual need. The activity tends to continue until the need is met. If the satisfaction of the need is frustrated, the activity may be intensified or varied, but with the same end. Among higher organisms and man the development of the psychic apparatus allows for a psychological elaboration of the same process. If a need remains unsatisfied or appropriate activity is blocked, the affect of anger may be felt which may have the conscious mental content of a wish to destroy, break, tear, injure or kill, or no conscious content at all. The aim and the process are biologically determined, but the object or direction may be changed and no connection between the biological and the psychological may be recognized. Thus one may see the whole or any fragment of the primary biologic behavior and its psychological elaboration. There may be preparatory changes in the musculo-skeletal apparatus, in the circulatory apparatus, in the gastro-intestinal tract or in the secretion of digestive enzymes, singly or any combination, with or without awareness of the meaning of these changes in terms of the affect of anger; or there may be any type of psychological representation of the affect, from conscious angry thoughts or phantasies, to all kinds of psychologic processes which delay execution of the act or which keep the affect or its object from consciousness, such as displacement, reaction formation, projection, turning against the self, etc., and with or without the above somatic concomitants. Again let it be emphasized that the biological process comes first in development, that phylogenetically and ontogenetically process and action precede the conscious awareness of their meaning. When examined from the point of view of evolution biologic processes as they appear in lower forms of life precede their corresponding representation and expression in higher forms. Freud's discovery of the unconscious receives confirmation in biology. The unconscious of each individual must have phylogenetic as well as ontogenetic sources.

And finally attention must be directed to the sexual instincts, the biological background of social relations, which tend more to serve species than individual survival needs, where at a new level the individual becomes subordinated to larger units, colony, herd, family, tribe or social group. Many different organisms end their life span when they have fulfilled their reproductive function and others die defending their young. We have already mentioned sexual differentiation into male and female and care of the young as two important developments consolidating the need for inter-animal relations. Again process and action precede awareness. Among the lower animals (and perhaps even the newborn human infant) inter-animal activities are purely biological. Wheeler brings numerous illustrations of this from observations of insects. The mature male moth initiates mating activities in response to an instinctually derived need for substances secreted by the mature female. Then with the aid of specifically sensitive chemoreceptors it is directed to the female. The presence of the specific substances on the female initiates the copulatory activity. Should the female be wiped with a cotton swab and removed the male will respond now to the swab. Among certain insects that take care of their larvae, secretions on the surface of the larvae attract the adult when the latter's need for the specific material reaches a certain intensity. While being licked the larvae obtain for food materials secreted by the adult during the licking process. When the need is satisfied, a new need develops leading the adult to return to the source of food for replenishment. In terms of the instinct concept we may say that an unbalance develops leading the animal to seek out the material which happens to be on the larvae, to be followed by a new unbalance leading the animal to return to the source of the nectar. No awareness by the insect of the meaning of this behavior need be postulated and any attempt to do so is nothing but anthropomorphism.

But among the higher organisms psychological representations of the same processes develop. The newborn infant relates to the mother through mouth contact and stomach activity in a fashion not much different from what we have just described. Ideally the mother responds to the nipple stimulation with pleasurable sensations and with contraction of the uterus. Pleasurable and unpleasurable sensations in the infant's mouth and upper gastroenteric tract are simultaneously in the service of nutrition and the mother-child relationship. With subsequent development, the biological and the psychological fuse, so that at the level of primary psychologic process all mouth and stomach activities are interchangeable. The same holds true for many other bodily processes, which simultaneously serve internal physiologic func-

tions and the requirements of inter-animal or inter-personal relationships. This is essentially the significance of infantile sexuality
and libido theory as described by Freud. With the development
of speech biological processes heretofore perceivable only as sensations of bodily change, internal or external, now achieve representation in a new form. Ella Freeman Sharpe[20] has demonstrated
how the metaphor, which depends so much on phonetics, can be
the verbal image of psycho-physical experiences of the preverbal
period. Further illustration of this view is found in Alexander's
vector concepts and in Lewin's[16] considerations of the oral triad of
wishes of earliest infancy, the wish to devour, the wish to be
devoured, and the wish to fall asleep, the translation of the earliest
biologic experiences of infancy into psychologic terms. Again we
discover biologic process and action preceding and circumscribing
the psychological expression thereof.

THE UNITARY CONCEPT OF HEALTH AND DISEASE

We may now return to Romano's designation of health and
disease as "phases of life, dependent at any time on the balance
maintained by devices, genically and experimentally determined,
intent on fulfilling needs and on adapting to and mastering stresses
as they may arise from within the organism or from without,"
where health represents a successful adjustment and disease a
failure. Our discussion so far amply supports such an interpretation and it remains now to elaborate upon it. Clearly health and
disease are relative concepts, so that at times no clear distinction
between the two is possible. This formulation takes into account
the processes existing between and within the total organism and
the total environment. The needs of the organism have a biologically determined source in instinctual energy, but satisfaction
of the needs is achieved through biological, psychological and
social devices. The aim is to maintain a condition of stable dynamic equilibrium between the internal and external environments.

How does failure of adjustment come about? Jennings, while
pointing out the essentially regulatory nature of the observed behavior of the lowest organisms, was astute enough to recognize
exceptions, that is, instances in which the behavior was not regu-

latory. His comments on this provide a good introduction to certain basic mechanisms whereby self-regulatory mechanisms fail. I quote:

"Without going into details, it is clear that there are a number of factors that would produce this result" (behavior that is not regulatory). "First, interference with the life process is not the only cause of reaction. The organism is composed of matter that is subject to the usual laws of physics and chemistry. External agents may of course act on this matter directly causing changes in movement that are not regulatory. Second, the organism can perform only those movements which its structure permits. Often none of these movements can produce conditions that relieve the existing interference with the life processes. Then the organism can only try them, without regulatory results, and die. Further, certain responses may have become fixed, in the way described above, because under usual conditions they produce adjustment. Now if the conditions change, the organism still responds by the fixed reaction, and this may no longer be regulatory. The organism may then be destroyed before a new regulatory reaction can be developed by selection from varied movements. This condition of affairs is of course often observed." Thus, even at the level of observed movements, it is possible to identify certain failures of adjustment in response to stress and to identify basic mechanisms.

We also need to consider at this time what constitutes a stress. A stress may be any influence, whether it arises from the internal environment or from the external environment, which interferes with the satisfaction of basic needs or which disturbs or threatens to disturb the stable equilibrium. Heretofore stresses have been conceived exclusively in terms of forces arising from the external world. Stress is relative, not absolute, since it depends upon the capacity of the organism to deal with any particular force at any particular time. As examples one might cite the different possibilities of effect of small pox virus before and after vaccination; of separation from the mother at the age of one year, six years, and 30 years; and of a sexual approach at six years, 15 years, or 30 years of age.

Further, as Jennings demonstrated in the most simple living

organisms, whether or not a situation is stressful depends upon the organism's past history, genically and experientially determined. Thus, the first experience may be stressful because the organism has not yet developed adequate defensive devices or does not have the endowment to do so. As examples one might cite the first encounter with physical agents such as bacteria when specific immunologic defences are not available; the child's first behavioral expressions of instinctual needs which conflict with the requirements of the environment as represented by the family; or the first requirements to assume adult responsibilities by a person who was greatly overprotected in childhood.

Or a subsequent experience may prove stressful because the earlier attempts at adaptation were relatively unsuccessful or incomplete, because the earlier adaptations are no longer appropriate, or because the first stress produced an unfavorable physical change. For example, one may respond to a second exposure to a drug or serum with a sensitivity reaction or to an operation with the revival of infantile complexes associated with separation or threat of injury.

In addition stress must be considered in a quantitative sense, taking into account both the magnitude and the time curve. How much, how suddenly, and for how long are important variables. There is apparently an optimal level of stimulation at each period of development leading to greatest adaptability, for both overindulgence and deprivation may disturb later capacity to adjust.

Claude Bernard pointed out that the conditions necessary to life are found neither in the organism nor in the outer environment, but in both at once. If we are to view disease as a phase of life, the same principle must hold true. While it is useful to categorize stresses as to their nature and relative importance, the concept of a single cause or stress in disease must be abandoned. Much more useful is the transactional point of view introduced by Bentley. Every dislocation of a stable equilibrium by a stress immediately introduces new stresses which may be more serious than the original stress and may require entirely different, and at times contradictory adaptive responses. One deals with a series of reactions of the organism in process with the environment. A complex mosaic of stresses is the result. It is nonetheless useful to consider stresses from three different aspects:

(1) The limitations of the organism itself, based on its physicochemical structure, its morphology, and the range of function of its parts and of the whole. For each individual one might identify the phylogenetic and ontogenetic determinants. They include the genic as well as the experientially determined limitations and potentials. In ways already described these factors will circumscribe as well as anticipate what will constitute stresses for any individual.

(2) Environmental processes, which interfere directly with the satisfaction of basic needs or which damage organs or parts of the body or disturb their function, thereby also interfering with the satisfaction of basic needs. These might include such things as inadequate food, water or oxygen, as well as inadequate love, disruption of an interpersonal relation, or the restrictions of a society; it might include physical trauma, parasites, poisons, etc. as well as the threat of these (i.e., physical trauma in retaliation for a forbidden aggressive or sexual wish).

(3) Changes in internal dynamics, which also necessitate a changed relationship to the external environment, such as occur during the various stages of the psychosexual development of childhood, during puberty, the menstrual cycle, pregnancy, the menopause, etc. Here the instinctual impulses themselves may acquire the character of stresses by upsetting the existing balance.

While useful at times, it is also however, arbitrary to specify the stress as primarily outer or inner in origin. More often we deal with a chain of events. For example, a virulent pneumococcus may produce not only pneumonia in the susceptible man but may also change his relationship to the external world in a number of ways which in themselves may be stressful to that individual as well as to other individuals in his social orbit. A sexual temptation or a provocative act by another person are examples of external stimuli leading to a change in internal dynamics. A change in internal dynamics may not only set in motion a whole new set of adaptive changes but may also provoke decompensation of a previously compensated somatic condition, as for example, when the anxiety reaction precipitates congestive heart failure in a patient with organic heart disease.

When a stimulus is encountered the organism must deal with it.

regardless of its source. If the capacity of the organism to deal with the stimulus is adequate, no disruption of equilibrium occurs and a state of health persists. If the stimulus cannot be dealt with, we recognize it as a stress which now upsets the previous homeostatic balance and disease is the consequence. If the stress is overwhelming the patient may die. Or a successful balance may again be achieved with no impairment of function, in which case health is restored, although the individual is no longer the same as before. Or a new balance may be achieved but at the price of considerable restriction of function, such as might be illustrated by a man with mitral stenosis who remains compensated if he limits his activity or the phobic patient who has no symptoms if he does not leave his room.

The clinical picture of disease, traditionally divided into symptoms, what that patient feels or complains of, and signs, what the physician observes by various techniques of examination, is contributed to by four components:

(1) The attempts at satisfaction of instinctual needs which have been interferred with. These may be simultaneously represented not only at biological, psychological and social levels, but also at different developmental levels (i.e., more primitive physiologic devices or metabolic pathways and more infantile psychosocial expressions). This is evident in the increased appetite and thirst of the diabetic, the air hunger of the cardiac, the call for help of the patient with pain, and the sexual symbolism of the hysterical conversion symptom. The biological, psychological, and social levels of expression of instinctual need is well illustrated by the case of a man with Addison's disease. Losing salt and water through the kidneys consequent to the adrenal cortical insufficiency he experienced a salt appetite to which he responded by the unorthodox behavior of surreptitiously drinking the brine from the pickle barrels in the delicatessen where he worked. When discovered and prevented from so doing, Addisonian crisis quickly ensued.

(2) The inner perception of a disturbed equilibrium or an unsatisfied need, involving the concept of a danger signal. This is anxiety, the signal alerting the organism to the threat of a

state of unpleasure or painful tension and setting in motion the adaptive devices to deal with this situation. The various systems of internal perception, unconscious and conscious, from chemoreceptors to the ego itself, are involved. If it achieves conscious representation, it may appear as feelings of anxiety, guilt, shame, remorse, as well as the more general feelings of malaise, weakness, fatigue, etc.

(3) The various adaptive devices, old and new, chemical, physiological, psychological and social which come into play to cope with the stresses, primary and secondary, to restore equilibrium and to assure satisfaction of instinctual needs. These may best be illustrated by an example, such as the invasion of a man by virulent bacteria. Here we see the specific and non-specific biologic responses to the bacteria, in the immuno-chemical reaction, the local inflammatory response, and the general change in bodily economy in the service of defence against the parasite. But we also see psychologic defences, illustrated by such phenomena as regression, increased dependence, withdrawal of interest in the outer world, etc., as well as defences against these, such as denial of illness, which may be required to deal with old dangers revived by the regression itself or by the fact of being sick or by the particular psychological meaning of the disease itself. And finally social means may be utilized in the struggle, such as recourse to available medical resources, hospital care, social agencies, etc. At times these attempts at adaptation may be in conflict, as when the dangers of a dependent situation lead the patient to deny illness or when the anxiety reaction with its physiologic preparation for flight increases cardiac failure. The largest part of the disease picture is contributed to by this complex interaction of the adaptive devices in the service of homeostasis.

(4) The actual structural or functional damage which may result from the stress itself (i.e., a scarred heart valve or a cavitation in the lung due to the tubercle bacilli) and from attempts at adaptation which are inappropriate or unsuccessful (ulceration of the duodenum secondary to excess gastric secretion; or edema due to retention of salt and water when the kidney responds to the failing heart as if the total volume of circulating blood was in-

adequate rather than simply the amount of blood reaching the kidney being inadequate; or atrophy of muscle and osteoporosis in the hysterically paralyzed limb).

From these four categories may be derived all the phenomena of disease. At times it may be difficult to decide in which category a particular manifestation belongs, but this is but an expression of the fact that each manifestation is over-determined. For example, the hysterical conversion symptom simultaneously expresses a wish (the instinctual impulse) and the defence against it (the attempt at adaptation).

Also we find that biological and psychological devices are to a considerable degree mutually interchangeable, a phenomenon which is phylogenetically and ontogenetically determined. The mental apparatus uses for expression and defences somatic systems which had been so used in the phylogenetic or ontogenetic past of the individual. The behavior of the organ or system so used is limited by its structure and function. Thus, the stomach may respond in the same way to a poison, foreign body or carcinoma as to a distasteful idea; it may manifest the same physiological response to a need for love as to a need for food. The biologic anlage of the basic types of psychologic response are found in unicellular organisms, to move toward, to move away from, to take in, to eliminate, to retain and digest, and to encyst. Alexander referred to the corresponding psychological behavior as vector quantities which are biologically conditioned and represent the fundamental dynamics of biological process. In man these tendencies are expressed through the appropriate physiological systems and in response to physical as well as psychological stress. It is probable that every system of the body participates in such reactions. The gastro-intestinal tract, the genito-urinary tract, and respiratory system, the skin, the sense organs, the circulatory system, the musculo-skeletal system, the endocrine glands, all have been demonstrated to respond physiologically to psychological influences. Recently Dr. William Greene[12] of our department in a psychologic study of patients with lymphomas, has provided some data suggesting that even the reticulo-endothelial system, functioning as a system of internal defence, may possibly manifest such indiscriminate responses.

The opposite relationship is also true. Physical changes in the body will have psychological representation. The perception of a swelling, of a disturbance in the body image, of a sense organ defect, indeed of any bodily dysfunction, may revive and make connection in the mental apparatus with residues of similar perceptions of a bygone period and perhaps having different meaning. The man who developed vasodepressor syncope when he suddenly discovered the presence of a hydrocoele is an example of such a process; a physical change mobilized early anxiety about mutilation.

It is manifestly impossible in this paper to do more than present a broad conceptual scheme. We have neither the time nor the knowledge to elaborate here all the varieties of unsuccessful adaptation, or to trace all the possibilities of contradiction between biological, psychological, and social adjustments. Much remains obscure and controversial and many chapters have yet to be written.

THE TASK OF MEDICAL SCIENCE

The unitary concept of health and disease helps to clarify the task of medical science. The physician must familiarize himself with and learn more about man's phylogenesis, both organic and social, and man's ontogenesis, biological, psychological, and social. He must understand man's basic needs and his means of adaptation in a physical, organic, and social environment. He must study the failures of adjustment and define more clearly their determinants and what constitutes meaningful stress. And finally he must study and devise new and more effective means of aiding the adaptive efforts of the sick patient. That many of the signs and symptoms manifested by the sick person are the attempts at adaptation and expression rather than the disease itself, as traditional medicine erroneously assumes, must be clearly kept in mind lest the attempt at therapy deprive the patient of defences without making more suitable ones available at the same time. This commonly happens in present day medicine when the specialist directs attention to one group of symptoms and ignores their significance for the total adjustment of the patient.

REFERENCES

1. ALEXANDER, F.: *Psychosomatic Medicine*. New York, Norton and Company, 1950.

2. BENTLEY, A. F.: Kennetic inquiry. *Science, 112*:775, 1950.

3. BERNARD, C.: *An Introduction to the Study of Experimental Medicine* (1865). New York, Macmillan Company, 1927.

4. BERNARD, C.: *Lecons sur les Phenomenes la de Vie Commune aux Animaux et aux Vegetaux*. Paris, Vol. 1, p. 50, 1878.

5. BERTALANFFY, L.: The Theory of Open Systems in Physics and Biology. *Science, 111*:23, 1950.

6. CANNON, W. B.: *The Wisdom of the Body*. New York, Norton and Company, 1932.

7. DARWIN, C.: *The Origin of Species by Means of Natural Selection*. New York, Modern Library, 1859.

8. DARWIN, C.: *The Descent of Man and Selection in Relation to Sex*. New York, Modern Library, 1871.

9. DARWIN, C.: *The Expression of the Emotions in Man and Animals*. (1872). New York, D. Appleton and Company, 1896.

10. DUNBAR, F.: *Psychosomatic Diagnosis*. New York, Paul P. Hoeber, 1943.

11. FREUD, S.: *An Outline of Psychoanalysis*. New York, Norton and Company, 1949.

12. GREENE, WM.: *Preliminary Observations on Psychological Factors in Men with Lymphomas and Leukemias*. To be published.

13. HALLIDAY, J. L.: Principles of Aetiology. *Brit. J. Med. Psychol., 19*:367, 1943.

14. JENNINGS, H. S.: *The Behavior of Lower Organisms*. Columbia University Press, 1906.

15. JENNINGS, H. S.: The Beginnings of Social Behavior in Unicellular Organisms. *Science, 92*:539, 1940.

16. LEWIN, B.: *The Psychoanalysis of Elation*. New York, Norton and Company, 1950.

17. MENNINGER, K.: Changing Concepts of Disease. *Ann. Int. Med., 29*:318, 1948.

18. ROMANO, J.: Basic Orientation and Education of the Medical Student. *J. A. M. A., 143*:409, 1950.

19. SEGUIN, C. A.: *Introduction to Psychosomatic Medicine*. New York, International Universities Press, 1950.

20. SHARPE, E. F.: Psycho-Physical Problems Revealed in Language: An Examination of Metaphor. *Int. J. Psychoanalysis*, 21:201, 1940.
21. SIMPSON, G. G.: *The Meaning of Evolution*. New Haven, Yale University Press, 1949.
22. WHEELER, W. M.: *The Social Insects*. London, Kegan, Paul, Trench, Trubner and Company, 1928.

V

ON THE ORGANIZATION OF PSYCHIC ENERGY: INSTINCTS, DRIVES AND AFFECTS

By

THERESE BENEDEK*

The idea of "unitary man," the theory of continuous interaction of the systems "world," "body" and "self," has obtained significant support from psychoanalysis. The basic structure of psychoanalysis—the instinct theory—in all its modifications represents the elaboration of the concept that there is a continuous energy exchange between the physical and physiological sources of stimulation and their derivatives within the psychic organization.

Considering mental life from a biological point of view, Freud defined instincts "as a borderland concept between the mental and physical, being both the mental representative of the stimuli emanating within the organism and penetrating to the mind and, at the same time, the measure of the demand upon the energy of the latter."[1] This definition is complex; it implies that instinct is a quantitatively measurable force "which compels the nervous system to complicated and interdependent activities."[1] It implies also that the quality of this force can be sensed and felt; that its fluctuations are accessible to insight and therefore can be studied by methods of psychology. Pointing out that the first meaning of the word refers to a sensual experience, Freud chose the term, libido, for the psychic representation of sexual energy. Thus, libido designates that quality of the instinctual force which can be felt.[2] Instinct, in general, represents an organization of psychic energy, the quality and intensity of which is felt as the

---

* Member of Chicago Psychoanalytic Institute.

impetus of a force driving toward the *object* (self or external) through which its aim can be fulfilled, its satiation can be achieved.[1] This definition of instinct coincides with the definition of drives. Is it then just a problem of semantic confusion, or the mistake of a translator* that the term, instinct, is used for the concept of drive? Or is there a meaningful distinction between these two concepts so that their clarification would be useful in further psychoanalytic research?**

Instincts—as the term is applied in Freud's theories—are not an identical concept with the instincts with which biologists deal in the lower species. They do not represent the rigid inheritance of the phylogenetic adaptations which set the limit to the adaptability of the organism. Since instincts in humans are subordinate to the principles which govern adaptive behavior, they cannot be considered as independent forces. Freud in his early contemplations assumed that instincts are subordinate to the "three polarities" which govern mental life as a whole. These are "subject—object" (i.e., individual—external world); "active-passive" and "pleasure-pain."[1] Freely formulated this means that the individual, being completely dependent upon the external world in order to survive, regulates his adaptive processes by the pleasure-pain principle.

The pleasure-pain principle is the indicator of the psycho-physiological equilibrium;[3] it announces the increase of psychic tension as pain and its decrease as pleasure. While it protects the constancy of the psychic energy, it also moderates the processes by which this stability can best be safeguarded. This principal regulator of the economy of the psychic apparatus has the power to coordinate all functions toward the aim of survival and for this purpose it can impel the instincts to participate in the adaptive processes. At a time when the ego is weak and its energies are not yet differentiated in articulate defense mechanisms, when an internal conflict or an external danger raises the psychic tension,

---

* The German word, Trieb, means drive, yet it is almost impossible to believe that Freud would not have disagreed with the translation if the English term "instinct" would have actually misrepresented his concept.

** The term "instinctual drive" combines the two terms indicating that these drives are more directly bound in the physiology of the organisms than drives, such as "drive for power," etc.

the adaptation may be achieved by a change in the instinct itself. Unconscious are the processes by which instincts may be repressed and they may change their directions, objects, and/or aims. Thus what Freud referred to as "vicissitudes of instincts" represents differentiations of instincts resulting from specific responses to various needs for adaptation. The adaptability of instincts is, however, not unlimited. After having participated in such radical changes, their adaptability reduced, the response pattern of instincts becomes more or less fixed. Thus through primary adaptive processes, the instincts participate in forming a pattern for the continual channelization of psychic energies. While this pattern is not completely rigid, it is characteristic for the individual; *it constitutes his personality.*

Personality, in general terms, can be defined as the individual's peculiar mode of dealing with psychic tensions. In other words, (from a dynamic view point) personality represents a system in which the psychic energies which participate in developing and maintaining the system are in continuous interaction with the energies which supply its actual functions. This is not a new concept. Freud, in developing his instinct theories, referred several times to an early proposition of Breuer, namely, that "there are two ways in which the psychic apparatus may be filled with energy" and that a distinction must be made between a "charging of the psychic systems with energy which is free flowing and striving to be discharged and one which is quiescent."[1,4] In accordance with Breuer's concept, we propose to recognize two phases in the organization of psychic energies. The psychic energy which participates in forming and maintaining the personality shall be referred to as *instinct,* whereas the term *drive* shall refer to the free energy which produces the current stimulation of the psychic apparatus.

Such distinction between instincts and drives appears to be especially useful at the present stage of our discipline when psychosomatic research directs our interests toward investigating the changes in the sources of psychophysiological energy.

It was the limitation of the psychological approach which led Freud to recognize early that the knowledge regarding the aims and objects of the instincts would out-distance in precision the knowledge concerning their source and intensity. While he awaited the investigations of the sources of instincts of other branches of biological sciences, he collected more and more data about the *quality of instincts*. These led him to the conclusion that the processes of life (for that matter, the continuous internal stimulation of the mental apparatus) are regulated by instinctual forces organized for acting in two opposing directions. Freud often reexamined his ideas about the instinctual regulation of psychic processes. His contemplations resulted in two major theories; in both of them he held fast to the dualistic organization of psychic energy.

As long as the aim of psychoanalysis was to divine the content of the unconscious and explain its role in the motivation of psychic processes and in behavior, it was satisfactory to regard the opposing forces as the *instincts of self preservation* and the *sexual instincts*. The instinct of self preservation supplies the energy for the functions of the ego; thus it was also called *ego instinct;* the sexual instinct, characterized by its specific affect quality, can be considered *libidinous instinct*.[2] The source of the instinct of self preservation (or ego instinct) was taken for granted as being the whole of the metabolic processes; therefore, it did not need to concern psychoanalysis. The source of the sexual instincts, however, concerned psychoanalysis, the more since their manifestations were attributed to an early age before the maturity of the sexual apparatus could account for them. In one of the shortest and most succinct presentations of libido theory, Freud states: "Sexual instincts are numerous, emanate from manifold organic sources, act in the first instance independently from one another and only at a late stage achieve a more or less complete synthesis. The aim which each strives to attain is organ pleasure. Only when the synthesis is complete do they enter the service of the function of reproduction becoming, thereby, generally recognizable as sexual instincts. At their first appearance they support themselves on the instinct of self preservation from which they only gradually detach themselves. In the choice of object also they follow the path indicated by the ego instinct."[1] Thus Freud indicated the anaclitic nature of sexual energy; the maturation as well as the function of the sexual instinct depends upon the processes which maintain the self, i.e., upon the manifestations of the ego instincts. In early infancy, there is a period during which only ego instincts—only physiology—is evident; then follows a period during which the developing libidinous energy appears fused with the energy of ego instincts. (The object of both is the same: mother—nourishment—self.) Only after significant developmental differentiation can the two types of instinctual energy be recognized as opposing forces. From that (developmental) time on, there exists an ever-present possibility of conflict between the opposing tendencies; these partake, in turn, in the further developmental processes of the personality.

The fusion and defusion* of opposing tendencies in the processes of development led Freud to induce a more comprehensive hypothesis which better accounts for structuralization of the personality and for the interchange of psychic energies. This hypothesis is known as the "theory of life and death instinct."[4] Although the concept of an instinct biologically urging toward death cannot be validated,[5] the vector concept** inherent in this theory has immense heuristic value. The antagonistic forces of this concept are the progressive *erotic instinct* which strives toward integration and the destructive *instinct of aggression*. Libido, in this frame of reference, loses its original meaning of a psychic energy which can be felt, experienced. It becomes psychic energy which functions unconsciously in integration, in fusion and defusion with its antagonist. In the same way, aggression is not only a psychic representation of the motor-energy in service of self preservation; it is a psychic energy which, through fusion and defusion with the integrative instinct, participates in the organization and in the function of the psychic apparatus. In the frame of this concept, the regulatory principle of psychic economy is not the pleasure-pain principle which can easily enter consciousness as affect. The economic regulation functions unconsciously as *"repetition compulsion." Fusion* of the originally opposing tendencies binds the psychic energy and achieves inte-

---

* This unusual term is applied in the English translation for the German term: *Entmischung*.

** Alexander in *Fundamentals of Psychoanalysis* refers to this theory as a vector concept.

gration in various degrees. If the psychic tension, so achieved, disturbs the stability of psychic economy, defusion is the process by which the component tendencies become free; from their independent energy-charge arises the need for discharge and/or for a new attempt at binding the antagonistic psychic energies. It is significant that these processes occur "beyond the pleasure principle" and that they are not accessible to consciousness.

The two instinct theories, successively developed, do not cancel each other. Each of these comprehensive theories retains its significance as the theoretical foundation of different aspects of mental functioning.

In the first place, the two instinct theories refer to two different phases in the organization of psychic energies. The second instinct theory affords the explanation of the basic processes. It implies that the instinctual energy originates in the physiological processes. While it is still obscure how the physiologic energy is transformed into psychic energy, Freud assumes that these processes constitute the id. The economic regulator of the id is the repetition inherent in the physiological processes. Psychologically, the processes of the id—the whole system of id—have the quality of the system Unconscious. The psychoeconomic regulation of its processes are the laws of the system Unconscious. It is the result of further integration of physiologic energies with psychic representations by which the id-energy reaches a phase at which the ego can experience it as originating in one or the other organ system; that one can *feel* it as hunger or as sexual need, as pain or as pleasure. When the result of the unconsciously proceeding instinctual organization brings about a psychic tension which is strong enough to pass the threshold to the *system Preconscious*, then the economic regulation is taken over by the pleasure-pain principle; then the integrative tendency of Eros may be felt as libido and aggression may charge hostile impulses. The preconscious phase of psychic functioning belongs to the realm of the ego. The preconscious processes still may remain qualitatively unconscious, i.e., unknown to the self, if the opposing, repressing forces of the ego exclude them from consciousness. The preconscious system is the sphere where the conflicting tendencies have their battleground and strive toward their particular aims. In these processes we recognize the conflicting instinctual tendencies of the first instinct theory: the opposing forces are then ego instinct and sexual instinct. Viewing it from the point of view of the permanent pattern of the personality, the first instinct theory seems to afford a frame of reference for that aspect of the personality—the self—which can be felt, which is accessible to experience. The second instinct theory offers the frame of reference for the organization and function of the psychic apparatus.

Freud arrived at this concept by studying primary organizations of the psychic energy such as the concept of primary narcissism and its differentiations, the organization of the ego's defenses and even more by investigating the interaction of the systems of the total personality: ego, id and superego. Psychoanalysts became so used to thinking in the frame of reference of organizational concepts that these systems often appear as existing "organs" by which the personality functions. Actually, these concepts refer to complex abstractions which, as such, cannot enter consciousness. Only their partial manifestations, particular id-impulses, special superego reactions (such as anxiety, shame, remorse) are accessible to experience. Whether we consider instinct as freshly produced id-energy, or bound organized psychic energy, it is through a *preconscious passage* that the instinctual forces achieve another level of organization and thereby become the motivating tendencies of conscious, goal-directed behavior and may enter consciousness as affects.

The principles of the transformation of psychic energy from unconsciously functioning id-energy to preconscious-conscious ego energy has been implicit in the metapsychological concepts of Freud. They have been restated in his posthumous work, *An Outline of Psychoanalysis*.[7] To this we add a terminological distinction when we refer to the former as instincts and to the latter as drives. Our contention is that this distinction has more than semantic significance, that it improves our methodology for investigating the interactions between somatic and psychic processes.

Many factors—physiologic and psychological—participate in the processes which regulate the continual exchange between the two phases of psychic energies. In the area of psychology, the laws of this communication are the same as those which determine the relationship between unconscious (id) and preconscious ego processes. Our contention is that the physiological factors which raise the level of instinctual energy to its preconscious state and influence its distribution and discharge in the ego (hormones, for example) are also accessible to psychoanalytic investigation.

Alexander's vector concept[8] has proved to be extremely valu-able in such an investigation. This concept refers to simpler biopsychological processes than the instinct theories. The three vector qualities of "intaking," "retaining" and "eliminating" repre-sent fundamental directions of biological processes. On their orderly sequence, life depends. Through them are the energies produced which supply the internal stimulation of the organism then to be integrated in the larger organization of psychophysio-logical forces. Alexander's proposition is that emotions, deprived of their ideational content, are the expressions of one or the other of these primary vector qualities. In the organization of the genital sexuality, the three vector qualities—the intaking, retaining and eliminating tendencies—achieve functional balance.* This concept permits further analysis of the sexual drive and reveals its components. Each of these components can be defined by its direction, aim and object; that is, each of these components has the characteristics of psychic energy and therefore they are re-ferred to as "psychodynamic tendencies." Since the psychody-namic tendencies represent a simpler abstraction than the more integrated drives, or the even more basic instincts, they offer access to the investigation of the changes in the sources of the sexual drive.

The psychoanalyses of the emotional manifestations in the course of the sexual cycle in women[9] offer a good example of the methodological significance of distinguishing the instinctual forces which participate in forming the personality and its structural

---

* It should be mentioned that the vector quality in Alexander's concept refers to function. The "surplus energy" which is responsible for the production of that "quality which is felt"—the libido—is beyond the single function and is produced by manifold processes from which it is, so to speak, filled into functions of other order, such as affects, emotions.

organization, from the psychic tensions created currently by the changes in the sources (or at least in one source) of the sexual drive.

When with the maturation of the organism the gonadal hormones take over the regulation and distribution of sexual energy, these find preformed patterns of psychic response and emotional discharge. This is in good accord with the concept of biologists. While hormones are absolutely necessary for completion of maturational processes which lead to procreation, "Hormone," quoting F. Beach,[10] "is to be regarded not as a stimulus to behavior nor as an organizer of the overt response but merely as a facilitating agent which increases the reactivity of the specific neuromuscular system to stimulation." What is "a genetically determined responsiveness of the nervous mechanism" can be equated with the response pattern of the personality in humans.

The study of the psychosexual fluctuations imposed by the gonadal hormones and/or the study of the gonadal hormones through the psychosexual manifestations has two intertwined phases. The first is that it has to consider the personality, its genetic, structural and psychoeconomic organization, in order to evaluate the influence which this relatively static system exerts upon the transient fluctuations of the psychosexual equilibrium. This influence is manifold. On this depends the ideational content of the emotions and affects, also the ego's ways and means of dealing with them; even more specifically, on this depends the quantity of libido which is available to fill the channels upon the various phases of (gonadal) hormonal stimulation. The other phase is the analysis of the day by day fluctuations in emotional expressions. Gauging the latter against the permanent motivation of the personality, the current emotional state and behavior can be interpreted in terms of the motivating psychodynamic tendencies. These, in turn, can be correlated with the qualitative changes and (relatively) quantitative fluctuations of the gonadal hormones. The high specificity of these correlations is evidence of the heuristic value of the vector concept.

Thus the study of the sexual cycle in women demonstrates the two phases in the organization of the psychic energy: that of *instincts* (energy bound in the personality) and that of *drive* which is stimulated by hormones. Since the sexual drive itself is highly organized, its component tendencies are revealed as the specific motivation of the emotional expressions related to the sexual drive.

However specific the psychodynamic tendencies may be, they too represent abstractions arrived at by analyzing the complex phenomena of emotional experiences. Of all psychic manifestations, *affect* is the one which most directly indicates the relation to the physiological source of stimulation.

Affect is a primary concept;* it indicates a feeling of or a response to a change in the psychophysiological equilibrium. Affect can be thus defined as that quantity of mobile psychic energy which has passed the barrier against stimuli and enters consciousness. "It is certainly the essence of an emotion, affect, that we feel it, that it enters consciousness."[6] Yet it is the system Unconscious (Ucs) where the affects originate. It has been pointed out before that it is in the system Unconscious where fusion and defusion, binding and freeing of instinctual energies take place. The origin of these energies is in the physiological processes. Thus *the system Unconscious is the relay station where the communication between physiologic energy and mental representations occurs.* The means of communication are the primary processes. The term *primary process*** designates a (relatively) free

---

* As far as psychoanalysis is concerned, affect has been the first concept of a psychic phenomenon charged with or having the task of discharging energy, which originated in the physiologic processes of the organism. Affect, however, is the forerunner of instinct, not only in the historical development of the instinct theory. Need and that which does away with need, its satiation, are primary affects; they are also considered as primary manifestations of instinctual energy. Pleasure of satiation, pain of need-tension, fear and anger are primary affects.

Since the structuralization of the psychic apparatus has become the main frame of reference of psychoanalytic thinking, the analysis of the affects has been neglected. E. Glover called attention to this fact in his paper, *The Psycho-Analysis of Affects.*[11] This as well as his later publications related to the subject have revitalized this primarily dynamic and phenomenological concept.

** We may consider different types of primary processes. Well known from dream work are the primary processes "in the mind" which produce the prelogical, dream-thinking, so different from the thinking of the wakeful mind. More pertinent to the problems of this paper are the primary processes of the instincts which are responsible for the vicissitudes of the instincts. They form a part of the "primary unconscious"; they enter into primary processes with memory traces of more recent instinctual occurrences and/or with psychic representation of *actual* physiological and mental processes.

exchange between the various elements of the system Unconscious. The most significant characteristic of the systems Unconscious is that the energy charges of its contents—whether they represent the physiological or the psychological aspects—are mobile in a much higher degree than in any other system of the psychic apparatus. Therefore, they can enter into primary processes in relation to each other. Through such transactions between physiologic energy and the psychic representation the instinctual force gains intensity. When it reaches the point where it activates the response of the pleasure-pain principle, this acts as a trigger which sets in motion further primary processes and brings about the affect.* The primary processes, like a kaleidoscope just shaken, produce a new Gestalt—affect—which the ego consciously perceives.**

Simple affects are the results of primary processes which relate the psychophysiologic energy and the mental phenomena which are its derivative. The latter enters consciousness as the ideational content of the affect. Often it is not the original affect which enters consciousness, but the one which is arrived at through mental elaboration of the first one and is remote from the first one by many steps. Sometimes such mental elaboration succeeds in diminishing the intensity of the original impulse; at other times the opposite occurs; often one affect mobilizes a whole cluster of affects which become more and more complex and are often accompanied by much alteration of physiological processes. (For example: surprise—blushing—embarrassment—anger at oneself because of that anxiety—crying.) Thus the unbound, free psychic energy overflows the barrier and sets the ego to the task of reestablishing the psychic equilibrium.

---

* The primary process itself binds a part of the psychic energy which motivated it and it may absorb so much free energy that none remains to overcome the barrier against stimuli; then the course of events remains unconscious and does not produce an affect. Unlimited are the number of simple affects which pass through the mental apparatus, leave their memory traces in the system Ucs and, holding it in a relatively mobile state, become a part of the adaptive apparatus; they may fulfill their function in exchanging their energy-quantities in primary processes without being felt.

** Freud conceived of the ego's conscious perception of what emerges from the Ucs as being similar to what the eyes perceive from the external world and convey to the cortex.

Can the study of such mental events reveal more about the physiological source of stimulation than we can learn by analyzing the ideational motivation of the affects?

"Affectivity manifests itself essentially in motor (secretory and circulatory) discharge resulting in internal alteration of the subject's own body without reference to the outer world," states Freud in one of his definitions.[6] Many investigations have dealt with establishing the parallelism between affect and its physiological accompaniment, yet these investigations deal with the external physiology of the affect-response rather than with the problem of the changes in the instinctual source of stimulation.

A simple relationship between instinctual stimulation and affect-response, however, can occur only in the new-born as long as no differentiation in the psychic apparatus has taken place. The first stage of mental life can be described as a state in which the fluctuation in quality and quantity of the "instinctual charges" may give rise to unmodified affect, i.e., the general motor discharge of the crying fit.[11] Just as unmodified is the response to satiation: sleeping. (Soon the infant has collected memory traces of the rhythmic change from need to satiation, memory traces of the touch of the nipple, the sensation of suckling, the touch of the skin; soon there appears the "expectation" of how the need should be made to disappear and somewhat later the first signs of object-relationship combine the need and its gratification with environmental influences.) As long as the ego has not yet developed defenses against internal stimuli, the affects arising from the body overflow the mental apparatus easily. We know but little about the affective experiences of little children, about the interaction between physiological sensations and the growth of the mental apparatus, between these primary affects and their representation in the psychic apparatus.*

The individual differences in the behavior of the new-born are only rarely considered as significant manifestations of the instinctual anlage, although they can be only a direct, unqualified

---

* In this respect, it is important to consider the effects of *pain* (for example, colic) for the development of the psychic apparatus; it may be that bodily pain prepares the mental apparatus for such radical adaptive processes as the "vicissitudes of instincts" are (e.g., masochism).

expression of it. There are, for example, great differences in suckling behavior. Some infants clasp the nipple with a biting grasp and suckle in a fast rhythm; their heightened excitement is obvious and often it takes quite a while until the greedy sucking calms down to the quiet rhythm of satisfaction. In some infants, such intense suckling activates pylorospasm or colic; others thrive well on it. For psychoanalysts, it is not difficult to imagine the dissociation in the emotional growth, when one considers the intense need to receive, to incorporate—and that this has been followed by pain, or even by vomiting, expelling the food. The need for relief, the desire for satiation, remain unfulfilled. Such an infant must miss in its development the security that need is followed by release, hunger by satiation. The memory trace of such experiences may be lastingly that of insecurity in regard to being satisfied. Therefore an anxious greediness may be the result even before object relationship develops and it may remain a lasting instinctual motivation of behavior.

Envy is a more complex affective manifestation of the receptive tendency than is greed, since it combines the receptive need with hostility toward the person who has what one wants. There is no doubt that the enhanced incorporative tendency of greed has an anxious quality: the fear of not being satiated is bound to it. Although the envy which the little child experiences is still a disturbing affect, its immediacy is diminished by the binding of the psychic energy. Thus the psychic energy, which originally charged such an unbearable need to incorporate that if it were not satisfied, the tension had to be discharged by crying fits, becomes bound in the mental processes of the personality; the envious child may sulk or may act out his hostility or may plan gratification (stealing), but may not cry under the tension of envy directly. During the further development of the personality, the painfulness of these affects compels various reactions and, by this, more and more of the original instinctual charge will be bound in object-relations and in other developmental processes, so that envy (or even greed) may become a structuralized part of the personality, a character trend. The envy of the envious individual, however, does not need to be conscious; it may be banned from consciousness by an effective superego. It may be disguised by overcompensation or other reactions; yet, under special conditions, the envy may be reactivated. An upsurge of a desire to receive, to own what someone else has, then recharges the original pattern of experience; envy enters consciousness and represents an acute affect with which the ego must deal. This crude presentation of the organization of envy is a relatively simple example of the complex affects. It serves here to demonstrate that psychoanalysis can follow the affect from the early manifestations of the particular psychophysiological need, which once diffusely took hold of the mental apparatus, through the repetitive organizational processes until it functions as a structuralized part of the personality. On the other hand, when envy, released from its restraint, enters consciousness as an acute affect, psychoanalytic observation accounts for the factors which reactivated the source of stimulation and thus mobilized the incorporative tendencies and hostility.

Generally, each complex affect can be analyzed in regard to (1) the psychodynamic tendencies which constitute it; (2) its genetic motivation; and (3) its function in the total personality.* To this is added the analysis of any disequilibrium in the psychic economy which brings the affect to the fore. There are periods when the envious person is not bothered by envy, a jealous person does not suffer from jealousy, the quarrelsome person appears conciliatory. Usually, external, environmental factors are held responsible for such changes. In the study of the female sexual cycle, it has been demonstrated that the variation in the psychophysiological equilibrium caused by gonadal hormones could also account for the individual's preparedness for a specific kind of affect-response. However, there are mood changes which may not be directly related to gonadal hormones but to other internal processes. Therefore, reliable methods should be developed to investigate physiological processes which direct the ego to perceive within the self, as well as out in the environment, those stimulations which incite the particular response.

---

* While the vector concept of Alexander is useful in analyzing the affects and emotions in regard to motivating psychodynamic tendency, his concept of emotional syllogism does not seem satisfactory for explaining the reactions to the affect which became a characterological, or otherwise functioning, part of the personality. The reaction formations originate from many sources; they are more complex than the emotional syllogism takes in account.

The source of simple affects is evident from the way they are brought about or are overcome (discharged). Tension-affects as well as discharge affects are felt and measured by means of the pleasure-pain principle, as well as by the observer's empathy. The reactive emotions which accompany need-tension (fear of frustration, sense of frustration, anger) as well as the reactive emotions to the affect of release (such as satiation, contentment, joy, elation) are motivated by the total personality and therefore they refer only indirectly to the change in the source of psychic energy. Thus, the personality as a whole determines the ego's conscious response to the affect and motivates the behavior. The ego's function, however, does not end there. The ego also perceives the phenomena of the behavior and integrates them as an *experience*. *"Erlebnis,"* or *insight,* which conceives the end-result of these integrative processes as "evident" as necessitated by internal forces even if it does not become aware of its steps, is accompanied by an affect of highest integration. Thus the sensation which gives the Erlebnis its quality of "being so," the quality of psychic reality, is a *mental affect.* Whether it conveys a conviction about one's own self or that of another person, this sublime accomplishment, too, is in the service of biological needs. Such mental affects are sharply contoured, isolated events which disturb the continuous surface of consciousness marking the need for and the ways of vigilance.

Consciousness is a condition of the personality, differentiated from the matrix of the system Unconscious with which it continually communicates. Affects of varying type and intensity produce oscillations in awareness and responsiveness, indicating that the organs of adaptation function by means of psychic energies freshly released from the reservoirs of instinctual energy. To trace this energy to its physiological sources and to follow its variations under social influence is the endeavor to which our science and this Institute is dedicated.

REFERENCES

1. FREUD, SIGMUND: Instincts and Their Vicissitudes. (In his *Collected Papers*, Vol. IV. London, Hogarth Press, 1949. Paper No. 4.)

2. FREUD, SIGMUND: *Three Contributions to the Theory of Sex.* Fourth edition, New York, Nervous and Mental Disease Publishing Co., 1930.

3. FREUD, SIGMUND: Formulations Regarding the Two Principles in Mental Functioning. (In his *Collected Papers*, Vol. IV, London, Hogarth Press, 1949, Paper No. 1.)

4. FREUD, SIGMUND: *Beyond the Pleasure Principle.* London, Hogarth Press, 1948.

5. SZASZ, THOMAS: On the Psychoanalytic Theory of Instincts: Evidence for a Unitary Instinct Theory. To be published in *Psychoanalytic Quarterly.*

6. FREUD, SIGMUND: The Unconscious. (In his *Collected Papers*, Vol. IV, London, Hogarth Press, 1949. Paper No. 6.)

7. FREUD, SIGMUND: *An Outline of Psychoanalysis.* New York, Norton & Company, 1949.

8. ALEXANDER, FRANZ: The Logic of Emotions and Its Dynamic Background. *Internat. J. Psychoanalysis*, 16:399, 1935.

9. BENEDEK, THERESE, and RUBENSTEIN, B. B.: *The Sexual Cycle in Women.* National Research Council, Washington, D. C., 1942.

10. BEACH, FRANK: *Hormones and Behavior.* New York, Paul B. Hoeber, 1948.

11. GLOVER, EDWARD: The Psycho-Analysis of Affects. *Internat. J. Psycho-Analysis*, 20:299, 1939.

VI

SOME ASPECTS OF MID-CENTURY PSYCHIATRY:
Experimental Psychology
By
David Shakow*

I have been asked to consider the relations of experimental psychology to psychiatry. Although the term "experimental psychology" has been widely accepted as "the psychology of the generalized, human, normal, adult mind as revealed in the psychological laboratory,⁹" such a narrow definition is now not justified, considering the breadth of modern psychology and the methodological ferment which characterizes it. I shall, therefore, deal rather with what I judge to be included within the spirit of the term, and trespass beyond the literal meaning by defining "experimental psychology" to be that psychology which is *oriented* to the laboratory and its controls, but which may be concerned with phenomena in non-laboratory situations where the attempt is made to achieve control of conditions. The "mind" may be animal as well as human, child as well as adult, aberrant as well as normal. The ensuing discussion will, I trust, provide the contextual body for this skeletal definition.

The statement has on occasion been made that psychology is the basic science for psychiatry in the sense in which physiology is for medicine. Although theoretically this may be justified and a reasonable hope for the future, evidence is not lacking for denying the actuality of such a status for psychology. Even traditional psychologists would, I believe, agree that psychology has not reached its promise of some half-century ago and has not achieved a codification of principles sufficiently broad to enable it to serve

---

* Professor of Psychology, University of Illinois College of Medicine.

as a sufficient foundation for any applied science or technology of *general* human behavior. (Its success in relation to certain specialized areas of human engineering based on knowledge in the fields of sensation and perception is, of course, outside our area of interest.[56])

Why is this so? The possible factors are many but this condition would seem to stem largely from the direction which psychology took in the second half of the 19th century on its release from philosophy—the direction pioneered by Fechner, Helmholtz, and Wundt, of a laboratory psychology modeled on physics and physiology, set up in the university tradition, and expecting to achieve sudden identification with the quantitative experimental sciences. Because of these special influences and the peculiar interests of the persons involved, psychology concerned itself with the microscopic and the segmental, especially with the fields of sensation and perception. Total life situations were almost entirely avoided, particularly in the area of the affective and motivational. Human-being-sensitive William James's natural reaction was to raise doubts about the contributions deriving from this approach and to insist that there were "more nutritious objects of attention" for the psychologist.

It is intriguing to speculate on what might have happened if instead of this laboratory approach, the French tradition of the hospital had become dominant, and experimental psychology had taken its start from experience there. Would psychology have a different face today? It took a "lonesome" person like Freud, working in the consulting-room by himself, to serve as a major force in counteracting this trend, a counteraction which did not, however, affect experimental psychology in any fundamental way until almost three-quarters of a century after its beginnings. Actually, as Bernfeld[8] has pointed out, Freud, through Brücke, was trained in the doctrines of the school of Helmholtz and Du Bois-Reymond, also fundamental influences on the early experimental psychology. Why did Freud and Wundt (by 24 years the older, it must be recognized), both brought up in physiology and medicine of a not-too-different kind, go such different ways in their psychology? Can it be that Freud, finding the academic path closed to him, was forced into extensive contact with patients, to become in the process the father of dynamic psychology, whereas Wundt could remain on in the academic setting of the laboratory, to become the father of experimental psychology? In the consulting-room Freud, despite, or perhaps because of, his scientific training was ready to deal with phenomena in the "intuitive" field heretofore the realm of the literary psychologist.[28]*

As Boring[9] indicates, general experimental psychology has had three historic phases in which the dominant problems were successively: (1) sensation and perception; (2) learning; and (3) motivation. Would experimental psychology be in a more advanced state today if these stages had been reversed? Or did the *Zeitgeist* just not permit such an order; especially a *Zeitgeist* aided by such powerful forces as Helmholtz and Du Bois-Reymond! The possibility, of course, exists that the particular kind of experimental stage through which psychology passed in the latter part of the 19th and the early part of the 20th century, a stage of a segmental, physical-physiologically oriented type, was a necessary step in the historical process of its development. Who can say? But certainly, the degree to which meaning and motivation were partialled out in the psychological study of the period and the great preoccupation with what was "pure," unfortunately resulted in a poverty, insofar as human and motivational problems are concerned, that only a tremendous intellectual revolution, such as is represented in Freudianism, could overcome.**

It should be pointed out that the intense "schoolism" in psychology of two and three decades ago is no longer a prominent feature of the present. The McDougall-Watson controversies of this earlier period have no counterpart now. Instead we find much more emphasis on experiments that have significance for various points of view, and considerable reinterpretation of fundamental approaches so that common factors, as well as differentiating aspects, are brought out. Disagreements among psychologists still

---

* What influence "act psychology" had on Freud, who had taken several courses under Brentano[39],[40] in 1874–6, is difficult to evaluate.

** This happened despite the influence of such persons as G. S. Hall, a most important figure in the psychology of the early part of this century. His advocacy of psychoanalysis apparently had little effect upon psychology. Freud's influence on psychology was at first indirect and largely exerted from without, through its effect upon the social scene generally, and upon psychiatry particularly.

exist, of course, but these are resulting increasingly in attempts
to reach understanding and to set up experimental tests of hypotheses.

It appears true, despite these advances, that psychology is a
self-conscious discipline. Because of its peculiar place in the
hierarchy of the sciences, situated as it is between biology and the
more strictly social sciences, and because of its not too remote
separation from philosophy, psychology has been preoccupied
with problems of methodology, and with self-examination generally, as reflected in its auto-historical interest. An unfriendly critic
could probably make a case for the neurotic character of some
of this self-preoccupation. He could point, for instance, to its exaggerated doubts, to the concern with techniques rather than with
content, to the too-ready imitation of the pattern and language of
the physical sciences. As against these characteristics, however,
one may point to the signs of developing maturity contained in this
pattern and to decided gains resulting from the process of self-
examination. The "neurosis," may I hopefully diagnose, appears
mainly to derive from natural adolescent needs and conflicts,
rather than from adult deviant needs.

Against this background, let us see what the preoccupations of
the psychology of the recent past have been, that may be of general or specific interest to psychiatry. In considering this topic,
it will be most profitable to devote the time to the area of methods,
attitudes, and approaches—that is, to an examination of how
psychology views its field and attacks its problems—and merely
mention in passing specific studies from some relevant areas of
psychology. The former area is especially important since psychiatry has many of the same methodological problems to solve.
I shall consider this topic from two points of view: the attitudes
with which a study is *approached*, affecting necessarily the way
it is carried out; and the methods that are used *after* a study is
completed. Since it will be impossible to mention more than a
limited number of specific studies, I shall consider them at appropriate places under method.

What kinds of questions are of special concern to psychologists
in approaching their material? Some prominent ones are: (1)
What is the primary subject matter of psychology? (2) What is

psychology's unit of study? (3) How should psychological studies be organized?

Throughout the history of psychology, different views have been held as to the nature of its fundamental subject matter. In the earlier years the range accepted for study was quite narrow. This century has seen a progressive expansion of what is included in systematic and experimental psychological investigation, so that at present the range of study is much broader, from simple sensory and motor processes through complicated social situations. Thus even so conservative a volume as the recent *Handbook of Experimental Psychology*,[56] has the following major sections: Physiological mechanisms, growth and development, maturation, learning and adjustment, sensory processes, human performance.

The trend, to take but one example, is seen in the changing attitude towards unconsciously determined behavior. Although a notion of the unconscious is already to be found in Herbart and Helmholtz, experimental psychologists for a long time refused to deal with this area. Only after Freudian views had affected psychology through various avenues, was the construct of the unconscious as explanatory of a wide range of behavior accepted as legitimate material for study.

One of the troublesome problems relating to subject matter has been that of the "single case." Allport[3] has expressed the conflict succinctly in asking the question: Should scientific law be taken to refer to "any uniformity that is observed in the natural order" or should it be considered to involve only statements of "invariable association common to an entire class of subjects?" If prediction in science must by definition involve prediction across individuals, then it is clear that the single case cannot be considered proper subject matter. However, there have been some stout representatives of the point of view that the *individual* may have his own laws. If we accept Kluckhohn's and Murray's[27,35] neat characterization of an individual's personality characteristics, namely, that each person is in some respects like all other persons, in other respects like some other persons, and in still other respects like no other person, then laws in psychological science have to take account of phenomena at all of these levels:

(1) universal; (2) type; and (3) individual. It is in relation only to the last that controversy arises.

The distinction between the nomothetic and the idiographic[3] is only a more elaborate way of stating this fundamental problem. The nomothetic view calls for a discipline with uniform general laws, whereas the idiographic calls for a discipline interested in particular events or particular individuals. Under certain limited circumstances, prediction is certainly possible for the individual, such prediction being made on entirely empirical bases, involving no "intuitive" acts. Psychology would, therefore, appear to gain from using both of these approaches.

Accepting some agreement on the subject matter of psychology, the complexity which faces the investigator when he is about to attack a problem is generally overwhelming. Within the organism numerous questions such as that of the latent as opposed to the manifest, the purely psychological as opposed to the physiological, the historical as opposed to the contemporary, confront him. When problems in the organism are further complicated by the variations outside, in the culture and the environment, variations that are created by a multiplicity of interactions, it is obvious that effective systematic study at any one time must be placed within set limits.

The experimental psychology of the past *did* set itself certain limits. It solved the problem of complexity, as in the case of structuralism, by chopping up its subjects, or, as in the case of behaviorism, by highly over-simplifying the situation through what one critic[7] has aptly characterized as a "glorification of the skin" at the expense of the brain and central nervous system. Such solutions, however, have been unsatisfying to many twentieth-century psychologists, psychologists who held that these methods of attack evaded the issue by destroying the very subject matter with which they were concerned. In the reaction to such approaches there has been much talk of dealing with the "organism as a whole." It must be admitted that sometimes this talk has been quite loose and naive, being merely a reaction to the elementarism of the earlier period. At other times, however, it has stemmed from rigorously developed theory.

We are faced here with the dichotomy that has been set up between one approach characterized by such terms as segmental, elementaristic, atomistic, associationistic and molecular, and the other for which such terms as total, organismic, field, and molar are employed. Although the context in which the different terms in each of these categories are used sometimes have different shades of meaning, for our present purposes we can consider them synonymous. We are necessarily concerned here with a problem of degree, for the extremes of these positions can experimentally be nothing but absurd. The fundamental philosophies of the proponents of each are clear. The major point at issue is whether even simple processes can be fully described or validly explained, if dealt with in isolation from other processes. If psychology is heading in any direction, in the recent past it seems to have been traveling definitely in the direction of the *total* approach.

It is of interest to note the difference between what is happening in psychology and in other sciences. The trend in physics as indicated by Born,[10] is in the direction of atomistics. One should, however, bear in mind that physics is a science that has shifted from the remarkably experimentally controlled one- or two-variable situation to the highly *disorganized* complex situation that calls for an actuarial approach. However, a science much closer to psychology, namely, physiology, seems also to be heading in the direction of atomistics, witness Adrian's statement, "..... physiologists have always been eager to learn....from the physical sciences in the way of new ideas and instruments and at present these seem to lead to the study of the cell rather than to that of the organism."[2] The question is essentially that raised so clearly by Warren Weaver in his article on *Science and Complexity*:[60] How is science to handle the problems of "organized complexity...... problems which involve dealing simultaneously with a sizable number of factors which are interrelated into an organic whole," —the kinds of problems which are so characteristic of psychology?

I shall consider some of the suggestions that have been made by psychologists in recent years to handle this problem. These proposals reflect psychology's attempts to come to grips with the fundamental questions relating to method of attack necessitated by the nature of its data.

With the development of notions such as those I have described, it is not surprising that controversies over heredity *or* environment, and organism *or* environment have lost some of their force. The trend has been to accept a psychology that deals with phenomena which involve these forces in *interaction,* even if in inexplicable interaction, rather than to attempt the operationally difficult, if not impossible, task of disentangling the contribution of each. Field theory has taken on an increasingly important role in psychology,[31] as it has in biology.[61]

On the basis of the acceptance of the principle that complexity should be left relatively undisturbed and that closer contact should be established with the original phenomena, more and more attempts are being made to bring into the laboratory as nearly lifelike situations as possible.

This is to be seen particularly in the social psychological sphere where studies of leadership and group life,[35] the effects of frustration on social relations of young children,[63] and studies in group dynamics[33] have, by setting up controls such as matched groups and systematically varied conditions, brought complex functions into the laboratory for investigation.

Another approach that goes even further in this direction is that represented in *psychological ecology.* This method takes advantage of actual field situations for the study of psychological phenomena. Since the approach is naturalistic rather than experimental in character, the problem of the refinement of the investigator as instrument is especially important. An example of this type of study is to be found in the researches of Barker[5] and his group at Kansas. A small community, "Midwest, U.S.A.," has been selected as a natural habitat in which to study normal childhood development. One aspect of this study is to follow a child around for a day making a systematic record of his behavior which by various coding devices is made available for analysis.[6] Another example is to be found in Brunswik's[15] studies of perception in which a person is observed in his daily environment to see how he actually deals with perceptual problems. In some respects, the psychoanalytic situation partakes of the ecological in the surrogate sense that it is a relatively free situation in which the subject verbally (and non-verbally) reproduces both his present and past outer and inner experiences and interactions. The studies of counselling and psychotherapy of the Rogers group,[50] in which recorded interviews are made available for systematic analysis, also meet in some respects the requirements for ecological study.[*]

One other aspect of the problem of achieving "wholeness" and recognizing complexity might be mentioned. I refer to the increasing consideration that is being given to the place of the "intervening variable." This concept was proposed originally by Tolman,[59] who developed a molar approach after a growing dissatisfaction with the segmental stimulus-response point of view. It has now been adopted also by those more closely identified with the latter point of view, as the complexity of even rote learning is receiving increased recognition. Emphasis is here placed upon the fact that variables exist between the stimulus and the response, which play an important role in determining the response that is finally made. Whether thought of in terms of past learning, "the apperceptive mass," drives, or in some other fashion, the growing awareness of the importance of such "unobservable constructs"[**] and the efforts to define them by their effects, are playing a considerable role in theoretical formulations in psychology.

Having faced up to the complexity of the data in these ways and in others that we cannot take the time to consider, the task is then one of reducing the material to manipulable units. This reduction must not, however, sacrifice the fundamental nature of the material as did some manipulations of the past. Various methods have been suggested to achieve this end of which I shall consider a few.

One proposal emphasizes a preference for one area rather than another because of greater importance. Lewin,[32] for instance, asked the question: Should psychology study the homogeneity of the factors that *produce* effects which may be quite varied, that is, the *genotypical;* or, should it, rather, study the homogeneity of *end-results,* arising perhaps from a variety of factors, that is, the *phenotypical?* Concretely, for example, is it the symptomatic or

---

[*] Cf. Darling[16] for an interesting discussion of the ecological approach to the social sciences.

[**] Cf. MacCorquodale and Meehl[35a] on the distinction between hypothetical constructs and intervening variables. Tolman[59a] apparently now prefers to make the intervening variables parts of more general hypothesized models.

characteristic aggression, or the underlying cause of the aggression, whatever its manifestations, that deserves primary investigative consideration? Lewin was critical of psychology for having generally over-emphasized the phenotypical and neglected the genotypical. Although Lewin was primarily interested in the cross-sectional approach rather than the longitudinal one of psychoanalysis, a sympathetic relationship between the two systems may be seen in the mutual primary concern with the genotypical in personality.

A quite different proposal for achieving limitation is that of the deliberate reduction in the field encompassed. We see this most clearly delineated in Hull's[23] attempt to provide a model for system-making in the field of learning by the use of the hypothetico-deductive method. He sets up a "miniature system" in which he isolates from the variety of psychological phenomena in the field of learning a few interrelated variables in the field of rote learning, and attempts to give a logically rigorous, systematic account of these in great detail. These miniature systems have played a prominent role in the development of the physical sciences. The hope is that psychology can, after detailed application of such systems in small areas, bring them together into larger and larger systematic units. For the development of such a system, a sufficient number of quantitative experiments must be carried out so that functional relationships can be defined with some assurance and the inter-relationships expressed in mathematical terms.[21] Such attempts are now mainly limited to several sub-areas of learning, a field where some of the most systematic work in psychology has been done. Several other limited fields also offer possibilities in this direction.

Still another way of approaching the problem of limitation is that taken by the animal psychologists. These investigators, having accepted the principles of evolutionary progression, hold that at least in the present stage of psychology, it is important and even essential to study psychological phenomena in simpler organisms. Infra-human animals, they argue, provide, in addition to relative simplicity of mechanism, a short life span, and the possibility of knowing the life history as well as of controlling environmental situations with a great degree of rigor. From this method of attack, to mention only some of the more directly relevant studies for psychiatry, have come such investigations as those of Liddell[34] on experimental neuroses in sheep and other animals, Maier[38] on "abnormal fixations" in rats, Jacobsen[25] on learning in monkeys with prefrontal lobectomy (studies that provided the rationale for the prefrontal lobotomy work of Moniz), Harlow's[20] studies of learning and "learning sets" (studies devoted to the important problem of how animals learn how to learn), and Levy's[29] work with dogs. Some animal psychologists recognize the dangers of extrapolating from animal to human subjects because of the importance of cultural influences and the markedly disproportionate cortical development in the human; others do not see the risk as so great, even while admitting marked disjunctions in evolutionary progression.

Another expression of the attempt to simplify the subject matter of psychology—a step, in fact, which goes beyond the mere limitation of the presenting field—is that seen in the points of view of psychologists like Skinner.[53] Without committing himself on the relationship between physiological and psychological phenomena, he holds that it is not necessary to concern oneself with physiological phenomena in order to understand the psychological data; psychological data, he says, should be dealt with in their own right. At the present stage of psychology, this is a defensible point of view which has the advantage of avoiding the neurological tautologizing which has been so prevalent in the psychological (and psychiatric) fields for many years.*

Although this point of view is held by a substantial group of psychologists, it should be pointed out, however, that there is another group, mainly physiological psychologists, who are strongly of the opinion that the concurrent study of physiological processes with the psychological is most important. In fact, some of them, mainly on philosophical grounds, hold the view that the physiological processes are primary and that "all psychological explanation must move in the direction of physiology."[48] A similar

---

* Rapaport,[48a] with a very different point of view from Skinner's, also recommends staying within the psychological realm, at least for the present. He proposes a psychological conceptual model based on psychoanalysis as being most inclusive of the observed phenomena.

point of view is put forth on theoretical grounds by Krech and Tolman. Krech[27a,27b,27c] argues that hypothetical constructs cannot be psychological and that in model-building, molar neurological events should be used. Tolman[59a] appears to have retreated from his earlier position[58] of opposition to neurological constructs and recommends the use of what he calls "pseudo-brain models," by which he means models comprehensive enough to meet psychological theoretical needs and not bound by present neurological knowledge. Hebb's[20a] recently proposed theory of behavior, based largely on neurological constructs, is an important contribution to the psychoneurological point of view. The majority of physiological psychologists, however, go about their *experimental* business, using *both* psychological (behavioral) and physiological concepts, apparently making the implicit assumption that they are dealing with phenomena at two different levels of emergence.

A characteristic of the recent period, too, has been an increased interest in studies of a longitudinal nature, especially with emphasis on the genetic.[26,36] It is also true, however, that certain groups (particularly the Lewinian), without denying the importance of the genetic, have systematically taken a point of view that emphasizes the importance of studying the dynamics of the existing situation, and therefore, have preferred a cross-sectional approach.[31] This has, of course, served as another way of reducing complexity.

We have considered rather briefly some of the problems connected with subject matter and with the definition of units of study. We may now turn to the problems involved in actually setting up a project.

In psychology, *experimental design* has become a matter of increased concern during recent years, largely through the influence of R. A. Fisher.[19] Because psychologists have been persistently troubled about how to handle with rigor the complex problems which they have to face, they have been much intrigued with the possibilities lying in the methods used by Fisher and others for planning and evaluating agricultural experiments. His procedures seemed to provide a way of reducing the expenditure of both the time and energy required in carrying through long series of single experiments on single relationships, through the adoption of designs which permitted a systematic attack on many variables at once, especially when supported by the statistics appropriate to such designs.

Closely related to this interest in experimental design is the growing recognition of the importance of *preliminary concept-ualization or hypothesis-testing* in experimental work. In the early part of the century, as a reaction to the then prevalent philosophical speculation and introspection, a marked antagonism to hypothesis and theory developed, resulting in a predominance of studies emphasizing "facts" and the accumulation of data for subsequent analysis. This probably reflected the similar trends in the physical sciences of that period.[14] Recent years have seen a definite retreat from this point of view, and increasing emphasis placed upon theory and hypothesis as a basic guide for both ex-perimentation and observation.

Another prominent recent development has been "operation-ism," the principle that concepts in science are to be defined in terms of the operations by which they are observed. Growing out of Bridgman's original formulation for physics,[11] and de-veloped for psychology largely by Stevens,[55] it has achieved recog-nition as a tool to be used *before* actual experimentation but *after* a scientific proposition has been made. It serves as a device for determining whether what has been said is empirically meaning-ful, thus aiding the experimenter to avoid pseudo-problems, prob-lems for which no observational test can be provided. The pos-sible misuse of the principle as an inhibitor of wider generaliza-tion, as well as other criticisms have been raised.[24] Instead of the exaggerated emphasis placed upon it at first, such cautions have led to operationism's falling into its proper role in the psychological scene as a device for increasing methodological rigor.

These are some of the problems faced before undertaking a psychological study. Two other developments during recent years, statistical analysis and factorial analysis, relate particularly to ways of viewing already collected data.

Because of the persistent cautions that experimental psycholo-gists have about their complicated material, there has been par-ticular receptivity to the controls provided by *statistics*. We have already seen the interest in the factors entering into the design and control of conditions under which experiments are conducted. Since the control ordinarily attained at this stage is only partial, psychologists recognize the need for using statistics to provide additional controls *after* the data are collected. This is achieved through partialling out factors not controlled before and during the experiment. In this area the *null hypothesis* has assumed considerable importance. The basic assumption is made that the experimental results under consideration arise from chance. It is then the obligation of the experimenter to disprove this hypothesis through the use of tests of significance and to show the degree of confidence which may be placed in the obtained results, that is, the degree to which they are *not* the result of chance. Aside from measures of sampling error, which are involved in the hypothesis, psychologists have used extensively other statistics describing the central tendencies and variation of groups, the inter-relationships between groups and among factors, as represented in the various kinds of correlation coefficients, and other procedures which modern statistics provide both for describing large and small samples, and for determining the dependability of differences.

Psychiatrists have at times been critical of this preoccupation with statistics by psychologists. This criticism has been justified on those occasions when statistics have been inappropriately used in certain clinical settings, when the stones of means and standard deviations have been substituted for the bread of clinical understanding. However, psychiatrists have sometimes shown a tendency to dismiss *any* statistical manipulation of material on general grounds. Such lack of regard for one of the really potent tools of science is a handicap to the development of psychiatry. Fortunately, this is beginning to be recognized. One of the contributions which psychology can perhaps make is a demonstration of the applicability of statistics to problems in the psychiatric setting.

Whereas statistics are used in order to deal with the inadequate controls of the experimental situation, *factor analysis* is used essentially to deal with the inadequately formulated concepts of the original experiment. It is a method whereby a set of inter-correlated performances are analyzed into independently variable factors. Thurstone,[57] one of the major leaders in this field, has pointed out that factor analysis is a powerful, but very definitely an *exploratory*, technique. It can be of great value in pointing up potentially profitable avenues to investigate. Factorial mathematical manipulation has, however, at times been substituted for preliminary rigorous psychological thinking-through of a problem. When used with carefully collected data, and with some systematic preliminary psychological hypothesization, it may in complex settings provide the basis for psychological insights not easily obtainable without its use. In the field of psychiatry, it has special appropriateness for the establishment of syndromes. Some attempts[17,43] in this direction have already been made, but these have not been successful because of incompleteness of the original data and lack of rigor in their collection.

Given this kind of a present-day psychology, a psychology that is concerned more and more with dealing with molar units in as controlled and quantitative a way as possible, what can we expect in the future, especially of that part which has the greatest relevance for psychiatry? The general goal can be no other than, in Adrian's words, to bring "the mind within the compass of natural science."[1] My own impression is that this will be achieved in a somewhat different way from that expected and hoped for by the founders of experimental psychology.

Psychology will probably increasingly model itself more directly on its nearer neighbor to the right, biology, rather than on its more remote neighbor in that direction, physics. At the same time it will recognize more fully its similarities to its neighbors on the left, the social sciences. In this way psychology will more adequately establish the proper balance between its capacities and its functions as a member of a scientific community that is so constantly faced with problems of ordered complexity.

I shall discuss the ways in which this trend will express itself under four headings: One relates to the unit of study, a second, to the conditions of study, a third, to inter-relationships in study, and the fourth, to the place of theory in study. In the course of the discussion, I shall also consider some special areas of investigation.

Let us take the first: *units of study*. I believe that the trend for the future will be a continuation of the interest in molar behavior, attempts being made to deal with larger and larger units of reaction. Instead of trying to simplify the organism by segmentalization, the organism will be permitted to react as a totality. "Simplicity" and analyzability will be achieved rather through improvement of the techniques of observation, through improved conceptual selection and analysis, and through improvements in statistical analysis. This is not to say that molecular study will not be continued as appropriate, and used fruitfully. In fact, it is very likely that molar study of the kind described will provide the basis for more reasonably oriented molecular study. What I am saying is that the psychologist will attack "cognitive-conative-affective" units, from which aspects of psychological behavior of interest to the experimenter will be partialled out for analysis. In this connection, too, I believe that the intensively studied individual case, for use in the determination of both general and idiosyncratic laws, will play a substantial role. It is, indeed, strange that nowhere in the literature is there to be found an adequately documented long-term individual record that would lend itself to systematic hypothesis-testing.

As another reflection of this point of view, we can expect that more studies will derive from real life situations. The ecological approach will provide data to be worked over by successive selective analyses from the total context of such threateningly detailed studies. To achieve this, techniques for making situations objective, such as films and specially trained observers, will be used to an increased degree. Is this not a return to a stage similar to the naturalistic era in biology? In a sense, it is just that. The naturalistic stage was glossed over in psychology. A reasonable case may be made for the proposition that psychology has sorely missed an intensive period of direct preoccupation with the bare facts of life, a gain to be obtained only from such an approach.

In association with the field studies, I would expect a further growth in the use of closer-to-life problems brought into the laboratory for more controlled study. In fact, the hope is that there will be a constant shuttling forth to the field to search for situations providing the relevant conditions not to be obtained in the laboratory, and back to the laboratory, to test out the field findings under more controlled conditions.

In relation to the second point, the conditions to be set up for the study of psychological phenomena, we can expect to see a development of greater objectivity in many directions.

We may anticipate an increased *"candorization"* of psychology, that is, the transformation of much more of what are now private and non-communicated data into public data, open for general examination. The range of phenomena transferred from the former category to the latter should be considerable. We have already seen a trend in this direction as relates to the study of the process of psychotherapy.[50] This will be strengthened in the direction of adding to sound recordings other revealing devices. Whether the implicit and the presently cryptic in behavior can be entirely brought to the public level is questionable, but that procedures and technical aids directed at constricting the private area considerably can be developed, is quite likely. Already available, although little used, are such techniques as the sound-film,[52] which make possible the recording of complicated behavior that can be made available for repeated individual and team study, and for systematic successive hypothesis-testing.

It seems inevitable that the clinical area will be placed under greater control, and even experimental attack. Experimental design will be improved and the statistical understanding of problems of a clinical nature will be increased. Such experimentation, I expect, will, however, be more productive than present and past experimentation because many more psychologists will enter this area of study *after* a substantial experience period in the clinical setting. Under such circumstances we can expect that experimentation and observation both in the laboratory and in the field will be more sophisticated.

An increasing trend towards *quantification* is to be expected, a quantification which will be appropriate, growing out of experience with complex psychological problems, rather than be the naive kind from which psychology has sometimes suffered in the past. Statistics and mathematical treatment of data appropriate to the complexity of the situation and especially appropriate to the individual are beginning to be developed and these should supplement other types of measurement. The application of various special correlational techniques such as "Q technique,"[54] probability sequence analysis,[42] and content analysis[51] are several promising developments in this area.

In connection with my earlier discussion of ecological studies, I should expect that the techniques of observation and the perfecting of the psychologist himself as a major instrument of investigation will show many advances. Considerable thought has in recent years been given to problems of this nature. We can expect studies of the experimenter himself to determine his capacities for accurate report, his biases and his other limitations. We can look forward to programs of systematic training developed to improve his span of apprehension and to refine him generally as an instrument. In this context, the place of psychoanalysis as a refining device must be thoroughly examined since its usefulness for this purpose is still controversial.

Apropos of the point about the individual case, which I made earlier in the discussion of molar trends, it is to be expected that psychologists here and also in the ecological sphere, will pay increasing attention to prediction. Just as prediction plays the leading role in astronomy, which is not an experimental science, so psychology, hampered so frequently from achieving satisfactory experimental control, should place more emphasis upon prediction for the validation of its findings. A beginning in this direction has already been made, particularly in the industrial field and even in some of the clinical activities of psychologists, but it is hoped that this area will see consistent expansion. From recorded predictions, and the bases for them, made as explicit as possible for subsequent check, a contribution of considerable magnitude, supplementary to experimental studies, may be made to the understanding of personality.

In the third area, that of the inter-relationships of psychology, the reference is mainly to the nature of the collaboration with psychiatry and other disciplines, but I should like also to mention team collaboration within psychology.

Since the major problems in this area appear to go beyond the compass of a single discipline, perhaps all but exceptionally talented and exceptionally prepared individuals can make their most effective contribution through joint effort. Here the logic of Weaver's[60] "mixed team" approach becomes obvious, and I should expect the future to show an increase in the amount of both intra-disciplinary studies of the kind exemplified by the Murray group,[45] and inter-disciplinary studies of which the Worcester[22] and Columbia-Greystone Associates[41] projects are relatively recent examples. The best inter-disciplinary studies, however, are likely to be those organized around concepts common to the fields involved. Through such joint research activities we can expect the development of the most effective communication between the disciplines interested in this area. Psychology, lying as it does, in the hierarchy of the sciences concerned with this problem, between physiology on the one hand and psychiatry on the other, is in some ways located at a strategic position to advance the process.

A necessary caution needs, however, to be expressed with respect to interdisciplinary activity. I have reference to the danger of achieving what Frankfurter[62] has called a "cross-sterilization" of the sciences rather than their cross-fertilization. This is especially to be feared in situations where sciences of different degrees of development, quantification, control, and status come into contact. Such deleterious effects are sometimes reflected in collaborative research projects where psychologists and psychiatrists, because of the lure of the exact and the simple, are drawn away from research on the less controllable and more qualitative psychological aspects of the problem to preoccupation with primarily biochemical and physiological material, the more quantitative fields of their collaborators. We might keep in mind what has at various times been suggested as a definition for maturity: the ability to tolerate uncertainty. In the fields of psychiatry and psychology the investigator has so many opportunities to exercise this blessed quality, that it is not strange if slips are more than occasional.

In the fourth area, that of the place of theory in study, one can expect an increasing trend in the setting up of theoretical models to serve both as bases for the codification of existing knowledge and as guides to further research. These can be expected to range from theoretical systems which deal in detail with small areas of study, e.g., Hull's[23] model for rote learning, to more ambitious attempts to deal with broad areas of science, such as is represented by the general theory of action.[45a]

I can only say a few words about the areas which I consider likely in the future to draw the particular interest of psychologists in the field of psychiatry.

One such area, of considerable importance for psychiatry, is the systematic study of normal persons. Psychology has during recent years shown a growing interest in the abnormal, neglecting somewhat the intensive study of the normal person, except as he is used for control purposes. Several investigations of normal subjects of which those by Roe[49] and Macfarlane[37] are examples, have impressed psychologists with the importance of giving the same detailed attention to the developmental and environmental factors in the personality study of normal subjects that has been devoted to disturbed subjects. The frequency with which pathological findings are to be found in persons making good and even outstanding adjustment leads to the obvious need for studying the stabilizing process. A larger number of psychologists having become acquainted with important personality factors and concepts through experience with the aberrant, a more adequate study of normal subjects now seems possible. The growing interest of psychiatry in mental hygiene and prevention should make such studies of direct value to psychiatry.

Two other areas of major interest to psychologists will, I believe, be research in psychoanalytic and other dynamic concepts, and in psychotherapy. With respect to psychoanalysis, it is to be expected that as intimate contact of psychologists with this field grows (and such contact has been steadily increasing in recent years) more and more experimentation on the theoretical postulates of psychoanalysis will be undertaken. With respect to psychotherapy, generally, it is to be expected that the relationship between the psychotherapeutic and the learning process will be systematically explored further; explored, I trust, on the basis of more thorough understanding and first-hand acquaintance with the complexities of psychotherapy. The impression cannot be avoided that many of the formulations offered thus far have been made on the basis of acquaintance with over-simplified forms of the therapeutic process.

Other areas of interest will perhaps be those of psychosomatics and somatopsychics which call especially for collaborative set-ups.

Still another area is that of nosology, where the proper use of factorial techniques based on adequate clinical data may result in a contribution of some importance. It is to be hoped, however, that the experimental psychologist's *major* concern in all of these areas will be to use the facilities for fundamental research on the problems of personality.

I have tried in broad outline to draw a picture of experimental psychology's methods and content, especially of the areas in psychology most relevant to psychiatry. As I look back on what I have written, I am impressed with how much more attention has gone to the consideration of method than to that of content.

The reason for this, I suppose, lies in part in the fact that in an essay of this kind, the presentation of contentual material requires too much unfair singling out of particular studies. Further, some difficulty arises in presenting even the selected studies in enough detail to carry sufficient meaning. Mainly, however, the emphasis stems from recognizing that at the present time even the best of studies in psychology are merely "gropings" toward the significant. The major significances at the present time seem rather to lie in the delineation of important areas for study, the asking of the proper questions, and the development of appropriate methods for attacking them.

It is customary to refer to the *youth* of experimental psychology, to talk of its infancy, or, when the optimist has the floor, its adolescence. Actually, is this true? Experimental psychology may be youthful in its *performance,* but is this also true of its *age?* We must recognize that experimental psychology is getting close to its century-mark. If we take that famous October morning in 1850, when Fechner, lying in bed, was struck with the solution to the problem of providing a scientific foundation for his philosophy—a solution which involved a quantitative relationship between bodily energy and mental intensity—as the birthdate of experimental psychology, then the century-mark *has* already been passed. With psychology's accomplishments during this period, we need merely compare those of chemistry which is only 50 years older, of organic chemistry which is 20 years older, or of biochemistry which is only half as old.

So it does not seem to be a matter of the passage of years (nor

of more gifted personnel, I am ready to contend!). I have sometimes toyed with the notion that the various sciences have their
own tempos of development, just as have the various biological
species. Maturity in different species, as we know, is reached at
quite different periods, the time for its achievement being roughly
correlated with the complexity of the species. Psychology's developmental tempo (and that of the social sciences generally) is
perhaps analogous to that of man, if the tempo of the physical
sciences is taken to be that of the dog, let us say. On some such
scale, then, what takes developmentally a month for physics would
take a year for psychology, a year would take a decade and a
decade a century. Comparing their respective spirals, the form
which perhaps characterizes best the path of progress,* the slope
of the spiral for physics would be steep, while that for psychology
would be quite gradual. If there is anything to this notion of
differences in developmental tempo, then we should perhaps be
somewhat less critical of the slow progress of experimental psychology. The impatience of a James in the 1890's,[46,114] which led
him to confront Fechner's accomplishments with little Peterkin's
pragmatic, "But what good came of it at last?," and the impatience
of a Broad in the 30's,[12,476] which led him to remark that psychology "has never got beyond the stage of medieval physics," should
be less cause for concern. For, by our new time scale, these came
respectively only three and seven years after the founding of experimental psychology! Although we can appreciate the impatience of these eminent critics as well as that of a society which
has such pressing need for dependable knowledge in this area, we
must be prepared for progress to be slow.

Fechner founded experimental psychology by contributing a
revolutionary notion—that of placing the *mind* under quantitative
experimental study. The persons who associated themselves with
this enterprise did not quite realize where they were heading
nor how complicated a task they had undertaken. But persons
who have successively taken up the battle, have continued working towards this goal stubbornly. Slowly and deliberately they
have held to experimental rigor, even at the cost of psychological

---

* Could we call this the "helical theory" of progress?

meaningfulness, to quantification at the cost of richness of quality, to impersonality at the cost of personality.

There have been psychologists, on the other hand, who recognized some limitations in this approach and who pressed for broadening activity at the cost of some temporary reduction in rigor. These have served as gadflies to the plodding oxen, not without a modicum of effect. Other social sciences that had no pretensions to being experimental or quantitative, having reached a stage of readiness for psychological enrichment, turned to psychologies which also had no such pretensions. Compare for instance the considerable absorption of psychoanalytic principles by cultural anthropology with the minimal effect upon it of experimental psychology.

Of course, in history's telescopic eyes, the fundamental point of view represented by this group of slow experimentalists may be correct, and in the end the wait may have been worthwhile. What one wants to be sure of, though, is that travel is along a *spiral* and not in a *circle!* Certainly, as one examines the work of at least some of the psychologists in this group, the latter appears to be the case.

Here the historian, who views development in the longer sweep, can be of help. As I pointed out earlier, Boring sees the history of experimental psychology as consisting of three phases in which sensation and perception, learning, and motivation were successively dominant. He has even gone so far as to say that: "The student of the history of psychology would not be promoting an absurdity if he placed on the horizon of his imagination three landmarks to represent the beginning of these three phases: Fechner's *Elemente der Psychophysik* of 1860, Ebbinghaus' *Ueber das Gedächtnis* of 1885, and Freud's *Die Traumdeutung* of 1900.[9]"

Certain developments in psychology in recent years have great importance for the understanding of these phases. As outlined by Boring, they were *successive* phases, separate and independent developments with little overlap among them. What we are seeing now is the growing recognition of the importance of the motivation phase and of the inter-relationships among the three areas. The period when learning was considered as merely cognitive and motor, and perception as merely cognitive, is rapidly passing. Instead recent years have evidenced a growing dissatisfaction with the studies of learning in humans as being *too* cognitive, a turning to learning in animals because of the possibility for studying in them really important motivating factors, and finally the penetration into the field of human learning of motivational factors, as seen in the concern with "emotional learning," and the interest in psychotherapy as learning.[18,44] Even more recently we see the invasion of the perceptual field by motivational problems.[13] Thus the early segmentalization into separate fields which grew out of a need for control, and which so dehumanized psychology, is now being replaced by a decidedly more integrated attack upon the organism.

We see then that even in slow-tempoed psychology there are signs of progress. The methodological activity which I considered in some detail earlier is still another sign. But the tempo of progress must be speeded up. Physics, having acted the hamster in recent years rather than sticking to its canine tempo, has made such a speed-up mandatory for the social sciences. Weaver's suggestions for dealing with the problems of "organized complexity" by the use of the mixed team approach and modern computational devices, have possibilities which must be exploited, as should those proposals I have mentioned as coming from within psychology itself. Above all, however, what an inevitably *adolescent* psychology needs, it is development by *mature individual* psychologists. This development should, of course, take place along the line of their own predilections, but accompanied by a recognition of the fact that at this stage of psychology's progress no promising methods, experimental, naturalistic, statistical, or other, and no theories or frames of reference, can be disregarded. What is needed is a greater tolerance for a wide range of approaches and a greater freedom from the rituals of science.[4]

Ralph Barton Perry, writing some 10 years ago *In the Spirit of William James,*[47] said of him: "Had he known the psychology of today, he would have said, 'The tent of psychology should be large enough to provide a place for the Bohemian and clinical speculations of a Freud, or the rigorous physiological methods of a Lashley, or the bold theoretical generalizations of a Köhler, or the useful statistical technique of a Spearman. Only time will tell which of these, or whether any of these, will yield the master hypothesis which will give to psychology that explanatory and predictive power, that control of the forces of nature, which has been achieved by the older sciences.' "

Some of us may take slight exception to the "Bohemian"; for the rest, can't we go along?

REFERENCES

1. ADRIAN, E. D.: The mental and physical origins of behavior *Internat. J. Psychoanal.*, 27:1–6, 1946.
2. ADRIAN, E. D.: Physiology. *Sc. Am.*, 183:71–76, 1950.
3. ALLPORT, G. W.: *Personality: A Psychological Interpretation.* New York, Holt, 1937.
4. ALLPORT, G. W.: The psychologist's frame of reference. *Psychol. Bull.*, 37:1–28, 1940.
5. BARKER, R. G., AND WRIGHT, H. F.: Psychological ecology and the problem of psychosocial development. *Child. Dev.*, 20:132–143, 1949.
6. BARKER, R. G., AND WRIGHT, H. F.: *One Boy's Day.* New York, Harper, 1951.
7. BENTLEY, A. F.: The human skin: Philosophy's last line of defense. *Philos. of Sc.*, 8:1–19, 1941.
8. BERNFELD, S.: Freud's earliest theories and the school of Helmholtz. *Psychoanal. Quart.*, 13:341–362, 1944.
9. BORING, E. G.: *A History of Experimental Psychology.* Sec. Ed., New York, Appleton-Century-Crofts, 1950.
10. BORN, M.: Physics. *Sc. Am.*, 183:28–31, 1950.
11. BRIDGMAN, P. W.: *The Logic of Modern Physics.* New York, Macmillan, 1928.
12. BROAD, C. D.: The "Nature" of a Continuant. In Feigl, H., and Sellers, W.: *Readings in Philosophical Analysis.* New York, Appleton-Century-Crofts, 1949, pp. 472–481.
13. BRUNER, J. S., AND KRECH D. (Eds.).: *Perception and Personality: A Symposium.* Durham, N. C., Duke University Press, 1950.
14. BRUNSWIK, E.: The Conceptual Framework of Psychology. Vol. 1, No. 10. *International Encyclopedia of Unified Sciences.* Chicago, Univ. Chicago Press, 1951.

15. BRUNSWIK, E.: *Systematic and Representative Design of Psychological Experiments.* Berkeley, Calif., Univ. California Press, 1947.

16. DARLING, F. F.: The ecological approach to the social sciences. *Am. Sc.,* 39:244–254, 1951.

17. DEGAN, J. W.: *Dimensions of Functional Psychoses.* Ph.D. Dissertation. Univ. Chicago, 1950.

18. DOLLARD, J., AND MILLER, N. E.: *Personality and Psychotherapy.* New York, McGraw-Hill, 1950.

19. FISHER, R. A.: *The Design of Experiments.* Sec. Ed. Edinburgh, Oliver & Boyd, 1937.

20. HARLOW, H. F.: The formation of learning sets. *Psychol. Rev.,* 56:51–65, 1949.

20a. HEBB, D. O.: *The Organization of Behavior.* New York, Wiley, 1949.

21. HILGARD, E. R.: *Theories of Learning.* New York, Appleton-Century-Crofts, 1948.

22. HOSKINS, R. G.: *The Biology of Schizophrenia.* New York, Norton, 1946.

23. HULL, C. L.: *Principles of Behavior.* New York, Appleton-Century, 1943.

24. ISRAEL, H. E., AND GOLDSTEIN, B.: Operationism in psychology. *Psychol. Rev.,* 51:177–188, 1944.

25. JACOBSEN, C. F., WOLFE, J. B., AND JACKSON, T. A.: An experimental analysis of the functions of the frontal association areas in primates. *J. Nerv. & Ment. Dis.,* 82:1–14, 1935.

26. JONES, H. E.: *Development in Adolescence.* New York, Appleton-Century, 1943.

27. KLUCKHOHN, C., AND MURRAY, H. A. (Eds.): *Personality in Nature, Society and Culture.* New York, Knopf, 1948.

27a. KRECH, D.: Notes toward a psychological theory. *J. Personal.,* 18:66–87, 1949.

27b. KRECH, D.: Dynamic systems, psychological fields, and hypothetical constructs. *Psychol. Rev.,* 57:283–290, 1950.

27c. KRECH, D.: Dynamic systems as open neurological systems. *Psychol. Rev.,* 57:345–361, 1950.

28. KRIS, E.: The significance of Freud's earliest studies. *Internat. J. Psychoanal.,* 31:1–9, 1950.

29. LEVY, D.: Experiments on the sucking reflex and social behavior of dogs. *Am. J. Orthopsychiat.,* 4:203–224, 1934.

30. LEWIN, K.: *A Dynamic Theory of Personality.* New York, McGraw-Hill, 1935.

31. LEWIN, K.: *Principles of Topological Psychology.* New York, Mc-Graw-Hill, 1936.

32. LEWIN, K.: Vorsatz, Wille und Bedürfnis. *Psychol. Forsch.,* 7: 294–385, 1926. (Reprinted as "Will and Needs," in Ellis, W. D., *A Source Book of Gestalt Psychology.* New York, Humanities Press, 1950.)

33. LEWIN, K.: The research center for group dynamics at the Mass. Inst. of Technology. *Sociometry,* 8:126–136, 1935.

34. LIDDELL, H. S.: Conditioned Reflex Method and Experimental Neurosis. In: Hunt, J. McV.: *Personality and the Behavior Disorders.* 2 vols., New York, Ronald Press, 1944, pp. 389–412.

35. LIPPITT, R.: An experimental study of the effect of democratic and authoritarian group atmospheres. Univ. Iowa Stud., *16:* 43–198, 1940.

35a. MacCORQUODALE, K., AND MEEHL, P. E.: On a distinction between hypothetical constructs and intervening variables. *Psychol. Rev.,* 55:95–107, 1948.

36. MACFARLANE, J. W.: Studies in child guidance: I. Methodology of data collection and organization. *Monogr. Soc. Res. Child Develop.,* 3: No. 6, 1938.

37. MACFARLANE, J. W.: Looking ahead in orthopsychiatric research. *Am. J. Orthopsychiat.,* 20:85–91, 1950.

38. MAIER, N. R. F., AND KLEE, J. B.: Studies of abnormal behavior in the rat. *J. Psychol.,* 19:133–163, 1945.

39. MERLAN, P.: Brentano and Freud. *J. Hist. Ideas,* 6:375–377, 1945.

40. MERLAN, P.: Brentano and Freud—A Sequel. *J. Hist. Ideas,* 10: 451, 1949.

41. METTLER, F. A. (Ed.): *Selective Partial Ablation of the Frontal Cortex.* New York, Hoeber, 1949.

42. MILLER, G. A., AND FRICK, F. C.: Statistical behavioristics and sequences of responses. *Psychol. Rev.,* 56:311–324, 1949.

43. MOORE, T. V.: *The Essential Psychoses and Their Fundamental Syndromes.* Stud. Psychiat. Psychol. Cath. Univ. America, Vol. 3, No. 3, 1933.

44. MOWRER, O. H.: *Learning Theory and Personality Dynamics.* New York, Ronald, 1950.

45. MURRAY, H. A., *et al.*: *Explorations in Personality.* New York, Oxford Univ. Press, 1938.

45a. PARSONS, T., AND SHILS, E. A.: *Toward a General Theory of Action.* Cambridge, Mass., Harvard Univ. Press, 1951.

46. PERRY, R. B.: *The Thought and Character of William James*. Vol. II. Boston, Little, Brown, 1935.
47. PERRY, R. B.: *In the Spirit of William James*. New Haven, Yale Univ. Press, 1938.
48. PRATT, C. C.: *The Logic of Modern Psychology*. New York, Macmillan, 1939.
48a. RAPAPORT, D.: The conceptual model of psychoanalysis. To be published.
49. ROE, A.: *A Psychological Study of Eminent Psychologists and Anthropologists and a Comparison with Biological and Physical Scientists*. To be published.
50. ROGERS, C. R. *et al.*: A coordinated research in psychotherapy. *J. Consult. Psychol., 135*:149–220, 1949.
51. SCHUTZ, W. C.: *Theory and Methodology of Content Analysis*. Ph. D. Dissertation. Univ. Cal., L. A., 1951.
52. SHAKOW, D.: The objective evaluation of psychotherapy. The evaluation of the procedure. *Am. J. Orthopsychiat., 19*:471–481, 1949.
53. SKINNER, B. F.: *The Behavior of Organisms*. New York, Appleton-Century-Crofts, 1938.
54. STEPHENSON, W.: The Significance of Q Technique for the Study of Personality. In: *Feelings and Emotions:* The Mooseheart Symposium. New York, McGraw-Hill, 1950, pp. 552–570.
55. STEVENS, S. S.: Psychology and the science of science. *Psychol. Bull., 36*:221–263, 1939.
56. STEVENS, S. S. (Ed.): *Handbook of Experimental Psychology*. New York, Wiley, 1951.
57. THURSTONE, C. C.: *Multiple Factor Analysis*. Chicago, Univ. Chicago Press, 1947.
58. TOLMAN, E. C.: *Purposive Behavior in Animals and Men*. New York, Century, 1932.
59. TOLMAN, E. C.: The determiners of behavior at a choice point. *Psychol. Rev., 45*:1–41, 1938.
59a. TOLMAN, E. C.: Discussion. *J. Personal., 18*:48–50, 1949.
60. WEAVER, W.: Science and complexity. *Am. Sc., 36*:536–544, 1948.
61. WEISS, P. A.: *Principles of Development*. New York, Holt, 1939.
62. WHITEHEAD, A. N.: *The Aims of Education and Other Essays*. New York, Mentor Books, 1949. (Intro. by Felix Frankfurter.)
63. WRIGHT, E.: The influence of frustration upon the social relations of young children. *Charact. & Person., 12*:111–122, 1942.

VII

THE BIOLOGY OF WISHES AND WORRIES

By

H. S. Liddell[*]

At a recent medical forum when discussion was in order, a physician arose and in a most deferential and mild manner said, "Mr. Chairman: May I launch a tirade?" I now make the same modest request.

Economics was called the dismal science when it sought to rob human behavior of its appropriate values. John Stuart Mill[1] long ago complained that the pursuit of wealth is impeded by man's "aversion to labor" and his "desire of the present enjoyment of costly indulgencies." Is psychosomatic medicine to become our contemporary dismal science? More than a decade ago John Whitehorn[2] wrote:

"The medical profession has a tendency to look upon emotion as morbid. Indeed, in recent years, so much is being said about pathological somatic conditions attributed to emotion, one might almost believe that emotions are to take the place of germs as the enemy in the next great medical campaign for health."

Today stress is the watchword. We have a physiology of stress, diseases of adaptation precipitated by enduring stress, and a stress sociology. Every morning one may hear on the radio morbidly oriented "good hints for good health" in which he is exhorted to perpetual vigilance about overweight, high blood pressure, cancer and the rest, and in the evening is challenged to establish regularity through the use of certain little pills.

In this pervasive atmosphere of tension and gloom to embark upon a discussion of the rational pursuit of pleasure may seem

[*] Cornell University.

an anachronism. It is almost as if one were to speak of the technique of playing the lute or the harpsichord. Nevertheless, I propose to consider pleasure—its biology, and its medical importance. To cushion the blow, however, I shall first speak briefly about the biology of wishes and worries.

During the past thirty years my professional life has centered uneventfully about the pasture and barnyard in the placid and friendly company of my experimental subjects, sheep and goats. In the late twenties while trying to repeat Pavlov's conditioned reflex experiments with the sheep I unwittingly precipitated an experimental neurosis in one of our subjects. The details of this chronic disorder of behavior in our sheep corresponded quite closely to Pavlov's description of conditioning neurosis in his dogs. Partly because of this laboratory accident our whole program of behavior study was reoriented toward the analysis of the stress factor in Pavlovian conditioning. Our previous studies of sheep and goat behavior had been concerned with the animal's ability to find its way through an out-of-door maze. Even when the sheep or goat was unable to learn its way through this labyrinth it remained placid and no nervous disturbances were at any time observed. However, when the animal was subjected to the restraint of the Pavlov conditioning harness neurotic disturbances became the rule during difficult or prolonged conditioning.

The simplest explanation of the sheep's placid acceptance of its inadequacy to learn the maze as contrasted with its neurotic breakdown when faced with a too difficult conditioning problem seemed to be a matter of initiative. In the maze the animal set its own tempo and could give up and lie down if it chose. In the conditioning harness the experimenter gave the signals at *his* pleasure and administered or withheld the appropriate "reward" or "punishment." The sheep, unable confidently to predict what was to happen next, could only "sweat it out."

For many years we have reversed the practice of "trying it on the dog." Training procedures intended for our animals are first tried on ourselves.

Let me try one on you.

I propose that each of you imagines himself to be a dog standing quietly but vigilantly, through force of habit, in the con-

ventional Pavlov restraining harness. To your cheek there is
cemented a simple device by means of which I may, at my pleasure, squirt into your mouth a small quantity of one-tenth per
cent hydrochloric acid. Now I am about to establish a trace
conditioned reflex to acid employing the tone of this pitchpipe
which I shall shortly sound. I shall sound the tone and after a
pause (which you are not to attempt to count off in seconds)
sharply tap on the table. You are to pretend that the sharp tap
is really the disagreeable experience of receiving a squirt of acid
in your mouth.

I shall repeat the test three times, beginning with a practice
run. The durations of tone and pause before the tap will remain
constant for all three tests. Ready! [Sound pipe 15 sec. Pause
30 sec. Tap.]

Now you who are sitting on my left close your eyes when I
tell you to, and those on the right will observe what you do. As
before, I will sound the tone and after the usual pause tap on the
table. Each of you with eyes closed, and with no counting to
yourself, will raise his hand when he thinks I am going to tap,
i.e., squirt acid in his mouth.

Ready! Close your eyes. [Sound pipe 15 sec. Pause 30 sec.
Tap.]

Once more. Those on my right act as subjects and those on
my left observe them.

Ready! Close your eyes. [Sound pipe 15 sec. Pause 30 sec.
Tap.]

I have often performed this experiment with classes and almost
invariably some subjects will hold in too long and at the tap fling
up their arms thereby releasing bottled up tension. I believe
most of you experienced relief or let-down at my tap.

Many of you, I suppose, have been thinking that in this make-
believe conditioning experiment nothing of vital importance to
you was involved and consequently it cannot give us much insight into the conditioned reflex experiments of Pavlov in which
his dogs participated in dead earnest. The hungry dog coming
to the laboratory has a keen appetite or, as Pavlov expressed it, a
passionate longing for food. The dog must similarly be in dead
earnest at the signal warning him that acid is to be squirted into

his mouth since this noxious agent threatens a sore mouth if many times repeated. His appropriate response will be to attempt to avoid the introduction of the acid by a jerk of the head or to dilute it, if it enters the mouth, by a copious secretion of watery saliva.

In our demonstration the sharp tap on the table was an incident of negligible biological significance. Yet Pavlov[3] discovered that under certain conditions the squirting of acid into the dog's mouth might also appear to be of negligible significance. The following remarkable experiment was performed in his laboratory. A trace conditioned reflex was established in a dog by sounding a tone for 15 seconds, and after a pause of 30 seconds acid was squirted into the mouth. (Our demonstration was in imitation of this experiment.) The sequence of tone, pause, acid was repeated 994 times over a period of one year and nine months. At the end of this gruelling experience the animal exhibited a remarkably stable trace conditioned reflex in which, from the beginning of the tone, approximately 25 seconds elapsed before the first indication of salivation appeared.

But now the dog was transferred to another experimenter who wished to establish a conditioned reflex of brief latency. In spite of random variations in the duration of the tone signal from 2 to 45 seconds with the introduction of acid always following immediately upon the cessation of the tone the dog persisted in his habit of precise delayed expectation and regardless of the duration of the tone the onset of salivation was always delayed 23 to 32 seconds from the beginning of the tone. For example in one day's experiment the tone was sounded four times for durations of 30 seconds, 2 seconds, 45 seconds, and 2 seconds. The negligible effect of the acid in the dog's mouth in eliciting reflex secretion of saliva was shown on the second and fourth tests of the day. In both cases acid was squirted after the tone had sounded for 2 seconds only. In test number 2 no saliva appeared for 29 seconds. This means that the irritating acid was sloshing around in the dog's mouth for 27 seconds but was ineffective in eliciting the appropriate protective salivary reflex. Again in the 4th test when the acid was administered at the end of the 2 seconds of tone the unconditioned salivary reflex arc remained unresponsive until 32 seconds from the beginning of the signal. Here the acid continued to stimulate the receptors in the mouth for half a minute without eliciting the reflex flow of protective saliva.

More remarkable still, when food was substituted for acid as the unconditioned stimulus or reinforcement the dog continued to adhere to his rigid and sluggish pattern of salivary response. When the tone sounded for 2 seconds and was immediately followed by food, the proffered food did not hasten the onset of salivation which still showed a latency of about 25 seconds. In other words, the food did not elicit the reflex secretion of the appropriate saliva necessary to make the bolus of food slippery for easy swallowing. These experiments from his own laboratory cast doubt upon Pavlov's conception of the primacy of the unconditioned reflexes in the organization of behavior.

In fact the whole conceptual superstructure erected upon such dramatic fictions as instincts and their survival value is called in question by observations such as those just detailed.

These simple experiments on animal behavior can, I believe, provide us with the essential biology of wishes and worries. No matter how passionate the hungry dog's longing or wishing for food, if he enters the laboratory situation where his wish must remain in a state of suspended animation (to suit the experimenter's convenience), in which he can do nothing to control the gratification of this passionate longing, then wishing becomes worrying.

Here one deals with the animal origins of the wish and of anxiety. But what can the experimental biology of behavior contribute to our understanding of pleasure? Psychiatrists, preoccupied with states of continuing pain and fear in their patients, have naturally and justifiably turned to the classical researches of Cannon and Pavlov for biological orientation. In this area of research the emphasis is on stress and bodily mobilization for emergency. The biology of relaxation and the pleasurable consequences of repeated success in the exercise of skills have, on the other hand, been relatively neglected. It is my opinion that psychiatrists are here taking the initiative in structuring areas of research which are about to undergo rapid development by physiologists and experimental biologists concerned with animal behavior. Two pioneers in this study are Sandor Rado and Thomas French.

Rado has introduced the fundamental conception of pleasure organization and French has been formulating a psychodynamics of needs and hopes.

According to Rado[4], man in the exercise of pleasure functions derives excitation from stimulating the sensitive spots available in his mind and body. These pleasure functions interact and combine with one another to make up to individual's entire pleasure organization. "The latter," he says, "is obviously neither sexual nor non-sexual, but an entity of a new order brought about by integration on a higher level. It undergoes typical changes during the life cycle, and is characterized at every stage by a measure of functional flexibility, working in the service of one and then another of the biological systems.—This pleasure organization requires a term that reflects its biological nature and avoids confusion between the superior entity and its component parts."

Music offers an illustration of Rado's thesis. The singer, for example, uses his breathing apparatus for aesthetic expression but in the case of the violinist the function of the motor mechanism of breathing is displaced to that exquisitely articulated structure, the bow arm. As every violin teacher tells his pupil, you must breathe with your bow. The typical changes during the life cycle mentioned by Rado are dramatically shown in the child's drawing. Here are seen the rapid rise and decline from the fourth to the twelfth year of a characteristic juvenile pleasure pattern. Doctor L. van der Horst[5] of Amsterdam writes, "In his drawing the child is influenced little or not at all by his elders. The adult hardly draws at all. The few who do so are too few in number to influence the development of drawing. However the ability to draw may develop at first, reaching its zenith in the puberal or prepuberal period; it subsequently fades, so that we are faced here with the precocious involution of a form of life expression."

During the past few years a fascinating study of preliterate deaf children from $2^1/_2$ to 5 years has been in progress at Public School 47 in New York. A colleague[6] who has participated in this study was impressed by the vitality of the urge in these children to develop pleasure patterns which seemed to compensate for their sensory handicap. For example, a little boy would experiment almost endlessly with rhythmic tactile patterns achieved by drawing a pointer over a row of vertical rods at different tempi. A little girl, on the other hand, made a pleasure ritual of washing the children's juice cups and luxuriating in the feel of the warm soapy water.

It is needless to mention the grave danger of anthropomorphizing when we observe animal behavior for evidences of the operation of a pleasure pattern. However, even so uncompromising a behaviorist as John B. Watson[7] in his *Behavior—An Introduction to Comparative Psychology* published in 1914 concludes his chapter on "The limits of training in animals" with these words, "Unsatisfactory as this chapter is from the standpoint of the strictly factual material it presents, nevertheless it serves to show that the behavior laboratories must be prepared to admit that the sympathetic upbringing of animals in the home where they are thrown into constant contact with human beings does produce in them a certain complex type of behavior for which the laboratory concepts as they now exist, are inadequate to supply explanation."

Perhaps, then, through a sort of emotional contagion our animal subjects and pets may be brought to the threshold of pleasure in skilled activity as we appreciate it and may exhibit in primordial form evidences of rudimentary pleasure patterns.

In concluding I shall refer briefly to Thomas French's[8] concepts of needs and hopes. He says, "As a first step toward the analysis of goal directed behavior it is necessary to make a distinction between two kinds of wishes. Many wishes arise out of unsatisfied needs. As examples of such needs we may cite hunger or pain, or fear. We may characterize the goals of such needs as negative. The wishes to which they give rise are wishes to get away from something. Such needs give rise to painful tensions which in the absence of other inhibiting factors tend to seek discharge in more or less diffuse muscular activity.—To such unsatisfied needs with their negative goals to get away from something painful or unpleasant, we may now contrast wishes that have been stimulated by opportunities for satisfaction or by memories of previous satisfaction. Such opportunities and such memories tend to give rise to hopes of satisfaction and to wishes to realize these hopes. The goals of such wishes are positive.—

"This distinction is important because of the contrasting effect of needs and of hopes upon the tension of unsatisfied desire. Unsatisfied needs tend to be experienced subjectively as feelings of unpleasant or painful tension. Needs increase tension but one effect of hopes of satisfaction is like that of real satisfaction. At least for a time hopes tend to relieve tension."

When the seige of Leningrad had been lifted I received from my friend, Professor Kupalov,[9] Director of the Pavlov Laboratories in the Institute of Experimental Medicine, his last letter before the iron curtain fell between us. He described a fascinating experiment which he was just undertaking.

The hungry dog (and, says Kupalov, the dog is always hungry) comes to the experimental room where through previous training he knows what to expect. In one corner of the room is a table A to which a door buzzer is fastened. When the buzzer sounds the dog jumps on the table and finds a portion of food. In another corner of the room is table B provided with a metronome set to click once a second. When the metronome clicks 60 per minute the dog jumps on table B and gets his bit of food. Placed on a shelf C on the wall is another metronome set to click twice a second. When this metronome sounds the dog finds food on neither table. The set procedure day after day is a signal from A, B, or C in random order but a signal is given every three minutes. The dog has no respite. Every three minutes a decision must be made. He must go to table A or to table B or if the metronome on shelf C clicks he is to do nothing since this is a no food signal.

After the dog has become accustomed to this monotonous and unavoidable procedure for some time, a small rug is placed on the floor in the center of the room. If he happens to be sitting or lying on this rug all signals will cease and he can take his ease. When he has learned to control his environment through the use of this rug he has an instrument of freedom.

Can we not discover such a magic carpet for ourselves? Perhaps even with our present limited knowledge of the therapeutic uses of hopes and pleasures we might safely predict that in many cases membership in an amateur string quartet might serve as a magic carpet and be more efficacious than ACTH, or that going fishing might be better therapy than cortisone.

REFERENCES

1. MILL, J. S.: *Unsettled Questions in Political Economy*, 1834.
2. WHITEHORN, J. C.: Physiological Changes in Emotional States. Research Publ. *A. New. & Ment. Dis.*, 19:236, 1939.
3. PAVLOV, I. P.: *Conditioned Reflexes*, 229, Oxford Univ. Press, 1927.
4. RADO, S.: Examination of the Concept of Bisexuality. *Psychosom. Med.*, 2:459, 1940.
5. VAN DER HORST, L.: Affect, Expression, and Symbolic Function in the Drawing of Children. *Feelings and Emotions.* Reymert, M. L., Edit., 398, McGraw-Hill, 1950.
6. CHURCH, J.: *Personal Communication*, 1951.
7. WATSON, J. B.: *Behavior*, 315, Henry Holt, 1914.
8. FRENCH, T. M.: Study of the Integrative Process: Its Importance for Psychiatric Theory. *Feelings and Emotions.* Reymert, M. L., Edit., 108, McGraw-Hill, 1950.
9. KUPALOV, P. S.: *Personal Communication*, 1944.

VIII

OBSERVATIONAL PSYCHIATRY:
The Early Development of Independent and Oppositional Behavior

By

DAVID M. LEVY*

When a baby is being spoon-fed at ten or eleven months of age, a mother is often delighted to find that baby grabs the spoon and tries to feed itself. Allowed to do so, he waves the spoon and spatters the food all over the room. Thereupon, the mother takes over, and tries to spoon-feed as before. It may happen that the baby will then purse its lips and refuse the spoon from any hand but its own. The mother's efforts in winning back the spoon, however persistent, may fail. Every variety of compromise then results, and peace is restored. In certain cases, however, the baby is adamant and accepts no terms at all, whether of partial assistance in handling the spoon, or in allowing a number of maternal feeds for a few of its own. The baby persists in refusal to accept the spoon from any hand but its own, and finally becomes sole possessor and manipulator of an instrument of feeding.

The baby's attempt to feed itself involved a struggle against the helping hand. Self-determined behavior of this type occurs long before it is put into words; the "I-do-it-myself" phase, so prominent at one and a half to two and a half years of age.

Self-determined behavior involves a struggle against the intruder as helper or as leader. For the parent, the most dramatic and difficult feature in the development of independent behavior is the "no! no!" or negativistic phase, in which obstinacy and

---

* Attending Psychiatrist and Psychoanalyst, N. Y. State Psychiatric Institute.

stubbornness and a clash of wills become the order of the day.

A two year old tries to fill the sink with water. He struggles to turn the faucet. His efforts are persistent, exhausting, and fruitless. His father waits patiently for a request for help. None is forthcoming. The father silently turns the faucet. The two year old bursts into a loud scream. He runs out of the bathroom. He is angry and in tears. He refuses to be washed or bathed. For him, everything is spoiled. An obstacle was thrown in the path of progress towards his own goal: his own job, to be done by himself alone, without the slightest help, or suggestion, or interference.

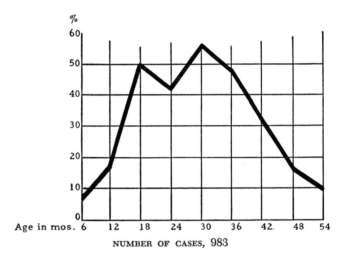

Age in mos. 6   12   18   24   30   36   42   48   54

NUMBER OF CASES, 983

In the process of maturation, besides the growth of skills, or better, inherent in the growth of skills, is the drive to master them. This drive which we observe as initiative, strength of response, and persistency, can be studied in various ways. It can be studied also in its social and non-social aspects; in terms, for example, of the drive exhibited in learning to creep, as well as the drive exhibited in opposing parental demands. In other words, it can be studied as skills and as attitudes.

The aspect of the early growth toward independent behavior that I wish to discuss on this occasion has to do with resistant behavior, as it is manifested within social settings.

My first illustration is taken from an investigation of the resistant behavior of infants and children during intelligence tests. Using the criterion of resistance, as the refusal to take one or more of a series of five tests, there appears to be a gradual increase in the frequency of this behavior up to a high point at 18 to 23 months, then a decline, and then another high point at 30 to 35 months. These peaks were found to be related to the sex distribution of the group, the female peak occurring at 18 to 23 months, the male peak at 30 to 35 months.

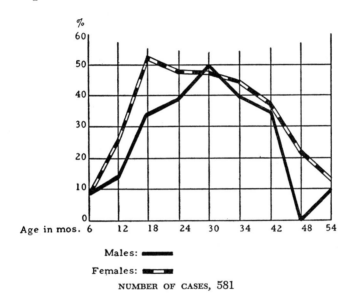

Males: ■■■■
Females: ■□■
NUMBER OF CASES, 581

This study of resistance was followed by a number of similar studies in this country. In Europe, the "resistant phase" became known as the "spite period" and was investigated along more clinical lines.

Of the American studies, I have selected one of a number as confirmatory evidence as shown in Table I, page 116.

The peak of resistance at 18 to 23 months has been confirmed a number of times. The sex difference has been confirmed by one other investigator. It was a consistent finding in six of seven distribution curves in our own studies.

Another method employed was the study of resistance during the physical examination in child health centers. Resistance was

TABLE I

Age Group	Refusal to take any test No.	%	Refusal of one or more No.	%	Total % refused
18–23	1	1.5	28	43.1	44.6
24–29	4	4.6	29	33.3	37.9
30–35	0	0.0	20	24.4	24.4
36–41	1	1.3	3	3.8	5.1
42–47	0	0.0	7	11.1	11.1
48–53	0	0.0	1	1.7	1.7
54–59	0	0.0	1	1.6	1.6

N = 506

From Stutsman, Rachel: *The Mental Measurement of Pre-School Children*, Table 21, p. 132, Yonkers, N.Y., World Book Co., 1931.

classified as type 0, no resistance; Type I, simple crying; Type II, some crying and struggling; Type III, crying and struggling to a degree severe enough to make the examination difficult, or impossible. An illustration is given of two curves of resistance, one

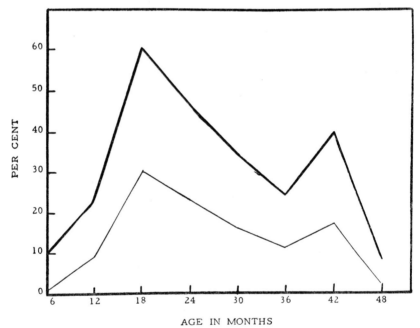

Resistant behavior during physical examination. Heavy line: Resistance Type II and III; light line: Resistance Type III. Number=624.

including Types II and III, the other of Type III alone. In this resistance curve as in others I have constructed, there is only the one high peak of 18 to 23 months. Why the second peak is no longer in evidence, I do not know. Possibly the intelligence test situation is a milder one than the physical examination, as a stimulus to resistant behavior. It elicits less aggressive behavior, and probably, therefore, makes possible a finer discrimination.

Another method consists of simple inquiry, questioning parents about the onset of the "no! no!" period and the onset of refusal to conform. The questions concerning the repeated use of "no! no!" and of "stubbornness" were asked in various ways, until they seemed to be understood, as verbal refusals and persistent non-conforming behavior. Regardless of the age of infant or child, up to and including five years, the vast majority of parents reported such responses as having their onset before age two years.

TABLE II

Onset of "No! No!" and Stubbornness

Age	Onset "No! No!"	Onset stubbornness
Less than 12 m.	4	4
12–17 m.	22	24
18–23 m.	14	12
24 m. or older	8	7
Totals	48	47

a. "No! No!" precedes stubbornness.......................... 29 cases
   In 20 cases, intervals 1 to 7 m.
   Median 6 m.
   In 9 cases, interval not remembered.
b. Same month... 8 cases
c. Stubbornness noted, "No! No!" phase absent................. 2 cases
d. "No! No!" not followed by stubbornness.................... 6 cases
e. Stubbornness precedes "No! No!"......................... 4 cases
Total .... 49 cases

Clinical studies also confirm these findings. The early histories of children referred because of oppositional behavior or for other reasons show similar progressions from a low to a high point. The differences lie in the intensity and duration of the resistant phase, rather than in its presence or absence. There may be differences also in the time of onset, since some highly oppositional children appear to be precociously stubborn.

Once the curve of resistance for a group is established, it is not difficult to test out various theories of resistance, when they lend themselves to the check of frequency or onset. Thus the theory that "only" children are much more likely to display resistant or oppositional behavior than children who have brothers and sisters, is not borne out by our findings. The percentage of type III resistance is about the same in "only" children and in children with siblings.

TABLE III

Resistance in "Only" Children
Aledo 1925   N = 123
Complete resistance indicated by*

Age in Months	No. Only Children	No. Children with Sibs
0– 5	I	III
6–11	IIIII IIIII IIII	IIIII IIIII III
12–17	IIII	IIIII IIIII III
18–23	IIIII II*	IIIII IIIII II*
24–29	IIII*	IIIII IIIII II*
30–35	I	IIIII* I*
36–41	III*	IIIII IIIII I* I*
42–47	IIIII I	IIII
48–53		I
54–60		IIIII II*

	N	R	%
Only Children	40	3	7.5
Other Children	83	7	8.4
All Children	123	10	8.1

It should be understood that these group studies have reference to groups; not to specific individuals. In any given case it may be quite true that highly oppositional behavior was initiated or intensified by a particular situation or cause, of "onliness," or a weaning trauma, or too early bowel training, or a maternal attitude. As a generalization, however, they may have little weight. My findings show no general relationship of early bowel or bladder training and resistant behavior. In the individual examples in my own practice in which bowel training appears to initiate negativistic behavior, the way it is done rather than when it is done seems to determine the sequence of events.

TABLE IV

Bowel Control and Resistance during Physical Examination.
One year olds.   N = 47

No. of Cases	Age in Mos.	Bowel Control	No. of Cases of Resistance Type				Percentage	
			0	I	II	III	II + III	III
17	12–15	Established	4	0	0	0	0	0
		Not Established	6	6	0	1	8	8
19	16–19	Established	0	1	4	1	83	17
		Not Established	3	2	5	3	63	23
11	20–23	Established	0	3	2	1	50	17
		Not Established	1	3	1	0	20	0

TABLE V

Bowel Control and Resistance during the Physical Examination.
2, 3, and 4 year olds.   N = 77

No. of Cases	Age Group	Bowel Control Established at	No. of Cases of Resistance Type			Percentage	
			0+I	II	III	II+III	III
8	2 yrs.	15 m. or younger	7	1	0	13	0
14	2 yrs.	16–20 m.	11	2	1	21	7
6	2 yrs.	21 m. or older	5	0	1	17	17
19	3 yrs.	15 m. or younger	11	3	5	42	26
5	3 yrs.	16–20 m.	4	0	1	20	20
6	3 yrs.	21 m. or older	5	0	1	17	17
7	4 yrs.	15 m. or younger	7	0	0	0	0
8	4 yrs.	16–20 m.	8	0	0	0	0
4	4 yrs.	21 m. or older	4	0	0	0	0
Totals (By age when bowel control estab.)							
34		15 m. or younger	25	4	5	27	15
27		16–20 m.	23	2	2	15	7
16		21 m. or older	14	0	2	13	13

One of the theories of the resistant phase has to do with the child's first use of the pronoun "I." The attainment of a word that involves a clear reference to the self results in a protest, it is thought, against the demarcation of the self from others, with consequent loss of support through dependency, and of feelings of omnipotence. It is an intriguing hypothesis, but the frequency curve of resistance does not support it.

TABLE VI

When Children First Use the First Person, "I"

Question asked at health station of 40 mothers, of 40 children, age range 12 months to 60 months.

29 reported that "I" was first used in speech at:

12 to 17 months in	2 cases
18 to 23 months in	6 cases
24 to 29 months in	6 cases
30 to 35 months in	4 cases
36 to 41 months in	4 cases
42 to 47 months in	3 cases
48 to 53 months in	4 cases

Of 29 cases where onset was recorded, it was 2 years or later in 21 cases.

In 8 instances, "I" was still not used in speech; ages of the children were 15, 20, 22, 24, 25, 31, 32, and 36 months.

In 2 instances, "I" was used but date of onset unknown.

The word, for most children, judging by our findings and the literature on this subject, comes later than 24 months, long after the onset and also after the peak of resistant behavior.

In clinical work, children are seen quite frequently because of negativism. The words used to describe them are stubborn, self-willed, defiant, mulish, spiteful, stiff-necked, oppositional, and many others. The adaptive nature of oppositional behavior is readily seen as an essential part of the process of growth in self-reliance, in self-determination. It involves a liberation from the first full dependencies and the full compliance that is their social counterpart. The freedom from that state is determined by mother and baby alike. The latter strains at the leash, the former loosens the bond. It is not an easy process, and a clash of wills is sometimes hard to avoid. It is difficult for parents to realize that extravagant display of oppositional behavior passes by, and the battle against it may do more harm than good.

When oppositional behavior becomes a main defensive pattern, it has a remarkably constricting effect on the personality; chiefly, I think, because it develops at the expense of spontaneity and affection. It congeals the individual, and though, in some cases, it organizes goal determined behavior quite efficiently, the triumphs are often empty.

The oppositional patterns may not be generalized. They may become limited to certain kinds of behavior, or to sectors in which negativism is particularly marked. I have referred to this type of negativism as "oppositional syndromes." Some children may show it particularly in school work; others in bowel refusals, in refusal to eat, or to wear an overcoat.

Oppositional syndromes may represent a holdover of defiance in unimportant areas of behavior. Starting along a special road of defiance, they may become, however, the early and main determinant of certain forms of intellectual inhibition, of anorexia nervosa, of obesity, of authority rebellion, and of a number of psychopathologic processes. The oppositional mechanism is unusually resistant to modification by psychotherapy, and deserves our special consideration, since the opportunity to modify it in childhood, once lost, may be regained, if at all, with great difficulty.

In the time at my disposal, I have tried to highlight, however briefly, some of the main problems in this field. Three questions that await further study might arouse your curiosity. Why the interval of one and a half years from the time of birth to the time when the maximal phase of resistance commonly occurs? How explain its recession? And what happens to those children who have no resistant phase at all?

Of more importance than these questions is the general concept of goal directed behavior, as it pervades the entire field of psychodynamics. The attainment of a goal which represents the culmination of effort and striving, may become so powerful a motive, in itself, as to be an oppositional and consuming force.

Besides directing your attention to this problem, I have tried also to demonstrate a method of investigation through data acquired by observation. The solution of many problems in psychodynamics has been attempted by building up a logical system on the basis of clinical inference. In solving a problem in psychodynamics, it is preferable to frame questions that call for pertinent observations, rather than dialectic.

IX

PSYCHOANALYSIS IN MID-CENTURY
By
M. Ralph Kaufman[*]

Psychoanalysis in the mid-century as a topic for discussion is an exceedingly complex assignment. It might, of course, be a didactic, schematic presentation which would fill in the details of the current systematization of psychoanalytic psychology. At the moment, however, it is more important to examine contemporary psychoanalysis from the point of view of those operational concepts in the foreground which seem most fruitful. The points made will be meaningless, however, unless they are seen in the terms and in the perspective of the psychoanalytic framework. This system has dynamic, genetic, economic, topological and structural aspects. In addition, one might at this time add the somatic aspect to this traditional metapsychological quintet of points of view. There have been recently adduced arguments justifying the inclusion of a somatic aspect.[32] Freud evolved the metapsychology as an indicator of the separation of his psychological investigations from the biological matrix out of which it had sprung. Recent studies in human biology, especially in psychosomatic medicine, and more precise observation of infantile physical development have furnished the biological data to which psychoanalysis can again return. This emphasizes that a mental event must also be described in terms of the physiological point of view,

[*] Psychiatrist to The Mount Sinai Hospital, New York City, and Clinical Professor of Psychiatry, College of Physicians and Surgeons, Columbia University, New York City.

I should like to express my appreciation to the various members of the staff of the Psychiatry Service of The Mount Sinai Hospital, and especially to Dr. Sydney G. Margolin, for helpful discussions which led to the form and content of this paper.

the consequence of which will be not only an advance of the frontiers of psychoanalytic knowledge, but also an indicator of the additional biological data that must be obtained. It should be emphasized that each of these metapsychological modalities can be both phylogenetically and ontogenetically viewed.

It is my intention to present for discussion only some of those fundamental concepts of psychoanalysis which are in the forefront of systematization at the present time. I shall try to correlate certain important contributions to basic theory with empirical data. Otherwise, this discussion would be a didactic exercise.

One of the problems in the forefront of our present-day discussions is the question of what is the essence of a systematization of human psychology that makes it psychoanalysis. There are certain basic postulates without which any system of psychology is not psychoanalysis, regardless of what else it might be. The central core of psychoanalysis is the concept of the Unconscious and of the various barriers involved in the process of a mental event becoming conscious.

Freud's instinct theory is of the utmost importance in activating this dynamic formulation. It is well known that there has been an evolutionary change in this theory. Originally Freud[7,13,15] postulated two categories of instincts—the sexual and the self-preservative. The latter he equated with the ego instincts. The empirical clinical observations which led to the hypothesis of narcissism[10] indicated that the ego was cathected by libidinal energy. As a result certain ego properties which have previously been in the service of self-preservation, of necessity, were aligned with the sexual instincts. In "Beyond the Pleasure Principle"[5] there was a restatement of another dual instinct theory in terms of the sexual and the death instincts. This development was a preliminary attempt to incorporate the aggression instinct by means of the metapsychological framework. Much controversy surrounded this step which has not as yet gained any great measure of acceptance. The current dualistic instinct theory tends to be limited to the sexual and the aggression instincts.

Freud's definition of an instinct is remarkable not only as a declarative statement, but also because it is an invaluable operational concept in research, theory and practice. It has been defined by Freud in a number of ways, one of which states,[12] "Instinct appears to us as a borderland concept between the mental and the physical, being both the mental representative of the stimuli emanating from within the organism and penetrating to the mind, and at the same time a measure of the demand made upon the energy of the latter in consequence of its connection with the body." He further stresses that an instinct must be defined in terms of its origin, impetus, aim and object. These factors, together with those having to do with somatic and mental properties, provide an extraordinarily large number of variables, which both singly and collectively enter into the definition of an instinct. As a result, the analysis of the role of a given instinct in any psychobiological process must yield explicit information concerning the quantity and quality of each of these properties. The method for this analysis, moreover, is implicit in the definition. For these reasons, Freud's instinct theory must continue to be regarded as a brilliant operational tool in psychoanalytic research.

The need to formulate a system of energetics within the psychic apparatus gave rise to the libido theory. Freud maintained consistently his psychobiological approach by pointing out that libidinal investment and libidinal shifts in the development of the personality were a function of maturational processes in the central nervous system and in the peripheral tissues of the body.[21] Some of these processes were influenced by specific experiences to which these bodily tissues were exposed in the progress of their maturation. The familiar example of this, of course, is his formulation of erotogenic zones and the progression of libidinal investment from mouth, anus and external genitalia. The instinctual drives, their manifestations and vicissitudes and their relationship to character structure, along with the biological thrusts in certain age periods, the concept of the infantile neurosis, the Oedipus complex, the so-called latency period are all interrelated and fundamental to psychoanalytic thinking. Recent physiological data based on experimental observations at The Mount Sinai Hospital[2,28,35] has furnished some powerful support to the libido theory in terms of the economics of the psychic apparatus and of the bodily responses to instinctual stimuli. There is a hypothetical tissue state which is the somatic aspect of the instinct as defined by Freud.[11] Hunger, thirst, fluctuations in steroid hormone metabolism and in other bodily chemical events —all are states of physiological tension which can be distinguished from their psychic representations in the form of appetite, thirstiness and such drives as sex and air hunger. The bodily states are regarded as hypothetical in that there is no scientific demonstration of the means by which these quantitative chemical changes create a tissue state which, of necessity, requires restoration to equilibrium. An aspect of this mental representation is manifested in dreams, free-association and day to day behavior in the life situation of the individual. Instinct and libido theories are valuable operational tools which help to orient research of this kind. For example, in order to show whether fluctuations in the functions of the stomach are due to hypothetical tissue states (hunger) or to its hypothetical mental representation (appetite), the formulation of a psychosomatically based instinct theory is required. It is by means of such considerations that such recent work as that of Mirsky, et al.,[36,37] Grinker, et al.,[24,38] Benedek and Rubenstein,[1] Margolin, Kaufman, et al.[28,35] and Wolf and Wolff[44] can best be understood. Margolin[33] on the basis of a review of recent work with ACTH and Cortisone suggests that a hint is afforded of the proof of Freud's statement[6,20] that chemical substances will be found which will function as the somatic substrate for the mental representation of an instinctual tension.

Instinctual aggression has assumed an important role in psychoanalysis as a basic dynamism in the total development of the individual and as a fused component of the sexual instincts. It is especially pertinent for the field of psychosomatic medicine. In a recent study on the psychophysiological varieties of aggression,[34] it was pointed out that the use of the term aggression to denote an event or a process in the mental life of an individual was a misleading over-simplification. It leaves out completely the profoundly important factors which are inherent in the concept of an instinct. In other words, in view of the fact that bodily processes and related psychic events are present at every instant, and since instincts are a complex of variables, many quantitative and qualitative varieties of aggression can result. As a consequence many different manifestations of varieties of aggression can occur, at times even simultaneously. Freud[18] in the context of anxiety stated an analogous problem in these words: "In describing the evolution of the various danger-situations from their prototype, the act of birth, I have had no intention of asserting that every later determinant of anxiety completely invalidates the preceding one. It is true that as the development of the ego goes on, the earliest danger-situations tend to lose their force and to be set aside, so that one might say that each period of the individual's life has its appropriate determinant of anxiety. Thus the danger of psychological helplessness is appropriate to the period of life when his ego is immature; the danger of loss of object, to early childhood when he is still dependent on others; the danger of castration, to the phallic phase; and the fear of his superego, to the latency period. Nevertheless, all these danger-situations and determinants of anxiety can persist side by side and cause the ego to react to them with anxiety at a later period than the appropriate one; or, again, several of them can come into operation at the same time. It is possible, moreover, that there is a close relationship between the danger-situation that is operative at a given moment and the form taken by the ensuing neurosis."

This discussion of the anxiety reaction illustrates the metapsychological handling of the concept. Structurally, as an alarm reaction in the ego which involves defense mechanisms; dynamically, as an illustration of a condition which indicates that a process arising from the id within the Unconscious has reached a nodal point at which it changes its position in the psychic economy, i.e., from unconscious it will become preconscious or conscious. Of the other aspects, economically and genetically, the latter is of especial interest because it illustrates the process which makes for the highly specific differences both in the stimuli and responses among different individuals.

Another basic postulate, that of the Unconscious[8,9,14,19] has received universal acceptance. It is especially important to remember that the Unconscious in psychoanalysis has in addition to the dynamic and topographic significance special laws of function. The clarification of the primary process with its displacement and condensation, the concept of psychic energy and cathexis, the mobility of psychic energy, first discussed in relation to the dream, is of direct relevance to the utilization of the concepts Unconscious and Conscious. If properly understood, it becomes impossible to think of the system Unconscious in terms of more-or-less awareness, since the Unconscious has laws of its own, and only in the sense of these laws can one properly utilize this concept. Since the Unconscious contains the archaic and repressed, it retains the mental representatives of somatic stimuli. Experimental work in psychophysiology can only be interpreted in terms of this concept of the Unconscious.

As an outgrowth of the structural point of view formulated in the "Ego and the Id,"[16] increasing interest has centered on the ego as an organization and as an apparatus of the personality and has resulted in a series of new and meaningful observations which throw light on the function of the ego within the total personality. Instinct as such or a unit of libido as such are never apparent in pure culture. It can only be manifested in the form of a transformation which is expressed by an experience in the ego. The means by which these transformations take place are of utmost importance and a re-evaluation of the ego in relation to the mechanisms of defense was formulated by Anna Freud.[4] An attempt at systematization of this aspect of the problem has recently been made in a series of brilliant papers by Hartmann, Kris and Loewenstein.[25,26,27,29,30,31] Transformation of instinct is one of the ego functions. Expression through motility, speech and thinking with affects is another. Perception has to do with other topological factors—the Preconscious and Conscious. The tri-partite division into the id, ego and superego as structural aspects of inter-related personality functions has had an important effect both in practice and theory.

There has always been in analysis a constant integration of theory and practice. In a sense no theory, hypothesis or construct was retained by Freud unless it stood up in the light of his clinical experience. On the other hand, each new elaboration in hypothesis or theory was reflected almost immediately in practical application. Perhaps two examples would be illustrative. The speculation regarding the death instinct was immediately reflected in some analysts' practice and was accepted by them as if it were a proven fact and utilized both clinically and in formulation of theory. Another example, with a much happier outcome, is the attention drawn to the ego as a system. This, as has already been emphasized, led to the whole series of valuable observations, constructs and systematizations which has greatly extended the borders of our knowledge.

Another aspect of this situation of speculation and of hypothesis in the theoretical areas has sometimes resulted in seeming validation which has been extended into practice and which has resulted in turn as a basis for revisions of theory based on the original mistaken premise. Some of the dissension within the psychoanalytic group can be traced to this feed-back mechanism. Many of the so-called modifications tend to go back to early developmental stages in the history of analysis, which have already been abandoned. In a sense they are regressions to theoretical positions which seemed valid in the light of the then known data.

One of the most valuable contributions that might be made to psychoanalysis at this time, but not in this place, would be a genetic study of the various dissident schools within psychoanalysis.

With the gradual evolution of theoretical concepts and the broadening of experience and the increasing acceptance of psychoanalysis within psychiatry, medicine and the sciences, new areas and opportunities for observation, experimentation and therapy have arisen. These in turn have reflected themselves back on to the actual practice of psychoanalysis. There has been a broadened spectrum as to the type of patient now considered treatable and treated. Hospitals influenced by psychoanalysis and staffed by psychoanalysts are now treating psychotics and contributing to our knowledge about them. There is another area in medicine, namely, the field of psychosomatic medicine, to which psychoanalysis has contributed and from which it stands to gain. In this field, the Chicago Institute of Psychoanalysis has among others pioneered. In a sense this represents a direct return to the biological source of psychoanalytic thinking.

The test of data in relation to psychoanalysis is two-fold. The first, the contribution made to the field in which the data have been acquired and the contribution that that field makes to psychoanalysis. Historically, it might be said that analysis has tended to develop as a self-contained system, after borrowing rather heavily from the biological and physical sciences of its time. It is well known that psychoanalysis has contributed generously to many fields, especially to the social sciences—to anthropology, philology, sociology, education and so on. On the other hand, it is probably correct to state that until recently these sciences have not contributed to the same extent to psychoanalysis in the sense of advancing its frontiers in terms of theory, practice or validation of basic concepts to any major extent.

Recent developments within the field of medicine, such as the dedication of this Institute, tend to fulfill a prophesy of Freud's.[3,17] Modern human biology has advanced to the point where its data and observations can add to and extend psychoanalytic theory and practice. Of extreme importance is that such developments provide independent methods of verifying psychoanalytic data and validating its theories. This is proceeding in several ways, namely, the psychophysiological observation of infant develop- ment by Spitz,[42,43] Ribble,[41] Putnam,[39] Rank,[40] Fries,[22] and Senn from within the psychoanalytic field.

Psychoanalysis has a synthesizing function in science. We must ask ourselves how each observation can be incorporated and in- tegrated with our own basic concepts and not how to translate our basic knowledge into the foreign languages of other disci- plines. Glover[23] has suggested, with some merit, that basic con- cepts in psychoanalysis can be used as research instruments into those areas where direct observation is as yet not possible.

This Institute for Psychosomatic and Psychiatric Research and Training is made possible because of the revolution in the funda- mental concepts of psychobiology, achieved through psychoanal- ysis, and because of this it becomes the function of the psycho- analyst to contribute to its ultimate goal in the light of his own basic knowledge and to foreswear the easy paths of pseudo-sci- entific eclecticism which ostensibly take the "best" from all ap- proaches. Each new fact must be screened through the exceed- ingly complex multi-dimensional frame of reference which takes into account the dynamic, the genetic, the topologic, the struc- tural, and the economic aspects of Freudian psychoanalysis.

REFERENCES

1. BENEDEK, THERESE F., AND RUBENSTEIN, BORIS B.: *The Sexual Cycle in Women. The Relation between Ovarian Function and Psychodynamic Processes.* Psychosomatic Monographs III, Nos. 1 and 2, 1942. (I. The Ovulative Phase. II. The Menstrual Phase.) In: *Psychosomatic Medicine, I*:245 and 461, 1939.

2. BERNSTEIN, SOLON S., AND SMALL, S. MOUCHLY: Psychodynamic Factors in Surgery, reprinted from *J. Mt. Sinai Hosp., XVII*:948, March–April 1951.

3. DEUTSCH, FELIX: Studies in Pathogenesis: Biological and Psychological Aspects, reprinted from *Psychoanalyt. Quart., II*:225, 1933.

4. FREUD, ANNA: *The Ego and the Mechanism of Defense.* New York, International Universities Press, Inc., second printing, 1948.

5. FREUD, SIGMUND: *Beyond the Pleasure Principle.* New York, Liveright Publishing Corporation, 1950.

6. FREUD, SIGMUND: *Ibid.*, p. 83.

7. FREUD, SIGMUND: *Ibid.*, Fn. p. 83–84.

8. FREUD, SIGMUND: The Etiology of Hysteria, *Collected Papers,* Vol. I, London, The International Psychoanalytic Press, 1924, pp. 183–219.

9. FREUD, SIGMUND: A Note on the Unconscious in Psychoanalysis, *Collected Papers,* Vol. IV. London, Hogarth Press and the Institute of Psychoanalysis, 1946, pp. 22–29.

10. FREUD, SIGMUND: On Narcissism, *Ibid.*, pp. 30–59.

11. FREUD, SIGMUND: Instincts and Their Vicissitudes, *Ibid.*, Fn. p. 61.

12. FREUD, SIGMUND: *Ibid.*, p. 64.

13. FREUD, SIGMUND: *Ibid.*, p. 67.

14. FREUD, SIGMUND: The Unconscious, *Ibid.*, pp. 98–136.

15. FREUD, SIGMUND: The Libido Theory, *Collected Papers,* Vol. V. London, The Hogarth Press and the Institute of Psychoanalysis, 1950, p. 131.

16. FREUD, SIGMUND: *The Ego and the Id.* London, Hogarth Press and the Institute of Psychoanalysis, 1927.

17. FREUD, SIGMUND: *A General Introduction to Psychoanalysis.* New York, Liveright Publishing Corporation, 1935, p. 338.

18. FREUD, SIGMUND: *Inhibitions, Symptoms and Anxiety.* London, The Hogarth Press and the Institute of Psychoanalysis, third impression, 1949.

19. FREUD, SIGMUND: *The Interpretation of Dreams.* New York, The Macmillan Co., Third Edition, 1927.

20. FREUD, SIGMUND: *New Introductory Lectures.* New York, W. W. Norton and Co., Inc., 1933, p. 211.

21. FREUD, SIGMUND: *Three Essays on the Theory of Sexuality.* London, Imago Publishing Co., Ltd., 1949.

22. FRIES, MARGARET E.: The Child's Ego Development and the Training of Adults in His Environment, from *The Psychoanalytic Study of the Child,* Vol. II. New York, International Universities Press, Inc., 1946, pp. 85–112.

23. GLOVER, EDWARD: *Basic Mental Concepts: Their Clinical and Theoretical Value.* London, Imago Publishing Co., Ltd., 1947.

24. GRINKER, ROY R.: Hypothalamic Functions in Psychosomatic Interrelations. *Psychosom. Med., I*:19–47, January 1939.

25. HARTMANN, HEINZ: Comments on the Psychoanalytic Theory of the Ego, from *The Psychoanalytic Study of the Child,* Vol. V. New York, International Universities Press, Inc., 1950, pp. 74–96.

26. HARTMANN, HEINZ: Technical Implications of Ego Psychology, reprinted from *Psychoanalyt. Quart., XX*:31–43, January 1951.

27. HARTMANN, HEINZ, KRIS, ERNST, AND LOEWENSTEIN, RUDOLF M.: Notes on the Theory of Aggression, from *The Psychoanalytic Study of the Child,* Vol. III/IV. New York, International Universities Press, Inc., 1949, pp. 9–36.

28. JANOWITZ, H. D., HOLLANDER, F., ORRINGER, D., LEVY, M. H., WINKELSTEIN, A., KAUFMAN, M. R., AND MARGOLIN, S. G.: A Quantitative Study of the Gastric Secretory Response to Sham Feeding in a Human Subject, reprinted from *Gastroenterology, 16*:104–116, September 1950.

29. KRIS, ERNST: Ego Psychology and Interpretation in Psychoanalytic Therapy, reprinted from *Psychoanalyt. Quart., XX*:15–30, January 1951.

30. KRIS, ERNST: Notes on the Development and on Some Current Problems of Psychoanalytic Child Psychology, from *The Psychoanalytic Study of the Child,* Vol. V. New York, International Universities Press, Inc., 1950, pp. 24–46.

31. KRIS, ERNST: On Preconscious Mental Processes, reprinted from *Psychoanalyt. Quart., XIX*:540–560, October 1950.

32. MARGOLIN, SYDNEY G.: *Some Metapsychological Aspects of Psychosomatic Medicine,* presented before the Boston Psychoanalytic Society, Boston, Massachusetts, October 4, 1950.

33. MARGOLIN, SYDNEY G.: *Personal communication.*

34. MARGOLIN, SYDNEY G., AND KAUFMAN, M. RALPH: *Some Psycho-*

physiological Varieties of Aggression, presented before Panel on Psychosomatic Problems, at the mid-winter meeting of the American Psychoanalytic Association, December, 1950, New York.

35. MARGOLIN, S. G., ORRINGER, D., KAUFMAN, M. R., WINKELSTEIN, A., HOLLANDER, F., JANOWITZ, H., STEIN, A., AND LEVY, M. H.: Variations of Gastric Functions During Conscious and Unconscious Conflict States, from *Life Stress and Bodily Disease.* 1950. Vol. XXIX of the 1949 *Proceedings of the Association for Research in Nervous and Mental Disease,* pp. 656–664.

36. MIRSKY, I. ARTHUR: Emotional Factors in the Patient with Diabetes Mellitus, from *Bull. Menninger Clin., 12:*187–194, November 1948.

37. MIRSKY, I. A., KAPLAN, S., AND BROH-KAHN, R. R.; Pepsinogen Excretion (Ureopepsin) as an Index of the Influence of Various Life Situations on Gastric Secretion, from *Life Stress and Bodily Disease.* 1950. Vol. XXIX of the 1949 *Proceedings of the Association for Research in Nervous and Mental Disease,* pp. 628–646.

38. PERSKY, H., GRINKER, R. R., MIRSKY, I. A., AND GAMM, S. R.: Life Situations, Emotions and the Excretion of Hippuric Acid in Anxiety States, *Ibid.,* pp. 297–306.

39. PUTNAM, MARIAN C.: Case Study of an Atypical Two-and-a-Half-Year-Old, from the *Am. J. Orthopsychiat., XVIII:*1–30, January 1948.

40. RANK, BEATA: Aggression, from *The Psychoanalytic Study of the Child,* Vol. III/IV. New York, International Universities Press, Inc., 1949, pp. 43–48.

41. RIBBLE, MARGARET A.: *The Rights of Infants: Early Psychological Needs and Their Satisfaction.* New York, Columbia University Press, 1951.

42. SPITZ, RENE A.: Anaclitic Depression: An Inquiry into the Genesis of Psychiatric Conditions in Early Childhood, II, from *The Psychoanalytic Study of the Child,* Vol. II. New York, International Universities Press, Inc., 1946, 313–342.

43. SPITZ, RENE A.: Autoerotism: Some Empirical Findings and Hypotheses on Three of Its Manifestations in the First Year of Life, from *The Psychoanalytic Study of the Child,* Vol. III/IV. New York, International Universities Press, 1949, pp. 85–120.

44. WOLF, STEWART, AND WOLFF, HAROLD G.: *Human Gastric Function,* London, Oxford University Press, 1947.

X

STRUCTURAL AND FUNCTIONAL APPROACHES TO THE ANALYSIS OF BEHAVIOR

By

Thomas M. French[*]

I

In the early years of psychoanalytic investigation Freud concentrated his interest on the repressed and unconscious parts of the personality. He resolutely postponed study of the "higher" mental functions until he had thoroughly explored the Unconscious. Later he began to correct this one-sided orientation.

Especially his analysis of the structure of the personality has won wide acceptance in the psychoanalytic literature. Yet our use of Freud's structural concepts has not really corrected the original one-sided orientation. We tend to think too schematically about the Ego and the Id and the Superego, trying to fit our patients' material into a uniform mold, instead of observing and analyzing clinically both sides of our patients' conflicts and the attempts of the integrative mechanism to find a solution for them. In this paper I am raising the question whether we cannot find a more flexible dynamic approach to the study of the total personality.

When Freud[5] first studied the dream work he attributed the act of repression to a dream censor. This was one of his first structural concepts. The dream censor, he postulated, distorts and disguises unacceptable wishes so as to make them unrecognizable. At a time when he was not yet ready to study the repressing forces, this suggestive analogy with a political censorship personified and dramatized a hypothetical repressing agent

---

[*] Associate Director, Chicago Institute for Psychoanalyses.

and permitted him to postpone further analysis of the motives that activate the dream censorship.

Now that we are interested in the functioning of the personality as a whole, *the motives that inspire the dream censorship are just as important* to discover *as the motives that are repressed.* Yet the great suggestive value of Freud's analogy with a political censor has made it easy to take the dream censorship for granted. In the psychoanalytic literature it is astonishing how often we neglect to inquire critically in each particular case what motives are responsible for repression.

When we do inquire, we find that the motives for repression are by no means always the same. The dream censorship is neither a person nor an impersonal system of the mind. In each case it is a specific inhibiting motive, an appropriate reaction to the particular dream wish that is being censored. Probably it is based in every case on the disturbing consequences of past attempts to fulfil a similar wish. For example, an intense dependent wish may arouse protest from the dreamer's pride; or a hostile impulse may give rise to a guilt reaction; or a sexual impulse in a man may stir up fear of the father; or the same sexual impulse may lead to fear of rebuff from the mother figure toward whom it is directed.

When we now study the dreamer's reaction we find that it is more than an attempt to give disguised expression to the disturbing wish. The dream work must struggle somehow to reconcile the two conflicting motives. The conflict between them is a *problem* which the integrative mechanism must try to solve. For example, the dreamer's pride, threatened by a dependent wish, may react with compensatory phantasies of independence or achievement, or may try to conjure up a situation in which the dependent craving would not be too incompatible with self-respect. The dreamer whose guilt has been aroused by his hostile wishes may imagine himself unjustly treated in order to justify his hostility; or his guilt may demand appeasement by a phantasy of being punished.

On the other hand when we content ourselves with the notion of a dream censor which we do not further analyze, we can easily fail to recognize the problem solving activity that is hidden behind tangled chains of associations in the latent dream thoughts.

II

Freud's two successive reconstructions of the origins of the conscience are two classical examples of an analysis that tries to take account of all the interacting motives.

The first of these reconstructions was part of his elaboration of the concept of narcissism.[6] One form of infantile narcissism is a kind of megalomania: the infant likes to imagine himself omnipotent and perfect. Yet his actual helplessness and the criticisms of his parents make it impossible for him to maintain this illusion. He protects himself from disillusionment by attributing the wished for perfection to an Ego-ideal. The Conscience arises as a need to achieve this ideal in reality.

Later, supplementing this account, Freud derived the Conscience from the child's attempts to resolve the Oedipus complex.[7] In the Oedipus complex the little boy's ambition to be powerful like the father fuses with his desire to possess the mother sexually. Thwarted in this desire by his fear of castration by the father, he is driven to seek another way of identifying with the father's power. He achieves this goal by imposing on himself the father's prohibitions, threats, and punishments. The part of the personality that splits off thus to identify with the father's prohibitive role is the Conscience or Superego.

The inverted Oedipus complex also contributes to the formation of the Superego, since the little boy is thwarted also in his desire to be loved sexually by the father. When the Superego takes over the father's role, submitting to the restraints and punishments imposed by the Superego can serve as a substitute for gratification of the boy's feminine desire to submit to the father.

III

However, since the publication of "The Ego and the Id", we often use the Superego concept as we once did the concept of the dream censor. Instead of emulating Freud's method of analyzing an interplay of motives we personify the Ego and the Superego and use them as explanatory concepts that seem to make further analysis unnecessary. For example, we may say that the Ego accepts an Id impulse, is punished by the Superego, and submits to this punishment. By thinking of Ego and Superego as persons, we seem to "understand" their "behavior" by a kind of empathy.

Yet personifying the Ego or the Superego, instead of helping, tends to divert us from the task of analyzing the integrative functions. The Ego and the Superego are both complex mechanisms. When we personify them we ignore their complexity. In order not to be diverted from the task of trying to analyze complex functions into their component parts, it is better, instead of the Ego, to think of the integrative mechanism; and, instead of attributing an inhibitory reaction to the Superego, we should try to find out whether a patient is reacting with guilt, or pride, or fear of punishment, or fear of loss of love, or some other specific conflicting motive.

IV

Fortunately we do not always make such schematic use of Freud's analysis of the structure of the personality. I shall not attempt an extensive review of the literature but shall merely mention a few studies that call attention to particular kinds of conflict that we frequently encounter clinically.

In an early paper discussing the differences between child analysis and the analysis of adult patients, Anna Freud[4] called attention to the fact that the child's Superego can usually not be counted upon to inhibit disturbing impulses unless it is supported by prohibitions from the parents or from the analyst. Evidently in these children the process of introjecting parental prohibitions has not been completed; and the prohibitions imposed by the superego must therefore be reenforced either by fear of punishment or by fear of loss of the parents' love.

In many adult patients the process of introjection of parental inhibitions is similarly incomplete; and fear of punishment or fear of loss of love are often the dominant inhibitory motives, supplementing or even replacing guilt. For example, in our studies of bronchial asthma at the Chicago Psychoanalytic Institute[3] we found that asthma attacks are precipitated only by situations in which fear of estrangement (or separation) from a mother figure is the inhibiting motive. During periods when introjection of parental prohibitions was more successful the patients developed other symptoms, such as neurotic compulsions, but were free of asthma.

Alexander has devoted considerable attention to another motive that is often responsible for repressions and reaction formations. He has pointed out, for example, that feelings of inferiority on account of strong dependent needs are often reacted to with aggressive criminal behavior; the criminal is trying to prove that he is not soft but tough.[1] Later Alexander called attention to the fact that such feelings of inferiority often come into direct conflict with guilt feelings.[2] Guilt inhibits aggressive impulses and subdues a man into submissive attitudes; but such submissive impulses give rise to feelings of inferiority that drive him again into aggressive behavior.

In a recent paper Piers[8] has elaborated this contrast further, insisting on the distinction between guilt and shame. The word shame, which he uses in a somewhat broader sense than usual, corresponds to Alexander's "feelings of inferiority." Piers finds the essential difference between guilt and shame in the fact that guilt inhibits and condemns transgression whereas shame demands achievement of a positive goal. He adds a structural distinction between guilt and shame: Guilt, he believes, proceeds from the Superego, shame from the Ego-ideal.

V

In trying to understand the reactions of the personality as a whole our basic task is to reconstruct the problem that the integrative mechanism is struggling to solve. To illustrate this approach I shall next discuss a dream analysis:

The dreamer was a 46 year old married man under analysis by Dr. Helen McLean* for bronchial asthma. He worked in a railroad freight yard where, on account of his asthma, he was treated very indulgently. In the twenty-fifth hour of his analysis he reported the following dream:

---

* This case is reported in Part II, Chapter III, of the Chicago Psychoanalytic Institute's monograph on bronchial asthma.[3]

Boxcar, in a room or building, like in office where we work. Door open in boxcar. Switchman called my attention to it. We both walked over and opened door further. Full of all kinds of merchandise, all unpacked. I pulled out pad of paper, kind of cheap so I threw it back. Then picked up a lot of pencils, all No. 1. Then took any pad, said I might need it later. Policeman or watchman came in and asked if door was closed. I said no and closed it—felt guilty about taking this pad and pencils. All I remember.

As the patient woke up from this dream he was wheezing hard. He had to use adrenalin.

His associations were as follows: In his work the patient often had to inspect boxcars. When the door of a boxcar was open the switchman wanted a man to go with him as a witness that nothing was taken. When asked to inspect a car, they often teased by saying "Bring it into the office." The analyst inquired if the paper and pencils resembled the paper and pencils that the analyst used to take notes....The patient said "No," that the pencils were like those that the railroad furnished. "Maybe I wanted to write a letter," he added, "Maybe I do, to father or brothers....I only think about writing home but don't do it. Didn't see father or brother in dream, only the two men I work with, one a switchman, the other a watchman. Here I was stealing, felt guilty, felt he would think I took those articles."

I shall not take time to report the hours just preceding this dream, from which it is evident that the patient is reacting to his treatment by a woman as a temptation. In the dream text he tells us that he felt guilty. Apparently stealing pencils and a pad from a boxcar has been substituted for some sexual impulse that disturbs him.

If some analyst were so disposed, I do not doubt that he could force this dream into the pattern of a Superego reaction based on the Oedipus complex. The watchman is an authoritative figure who is calling the dreamer to account. The dream text also calls him a policeman. He might well be a projected image of the patient's Superego. If the analyst to whom the patient feels attracted is a mother figure he should feel guilty toward the father and it is therefore fitting that his Superego should be represented by a man.

However, this interpretation has not attempted to bring the details of the dream text and associations into relation with the dreamer's actual conflict situation. Who does the switchman represent? And what is the meaning of his showing the dreamer the open door of the boxcar? When the watchman appears he asks whether the door was closed. What is the meaning of this question?

To understand these details we must reconstruct the patient's conflict more carefully. He is probably reacting not only to the seductive implications of being alone with a woman but also to the permissiveness of the therapeutic situation. In the therapeutic situation he is encouraged to talk freely even about forbidden topics. The open door of the boxcar symbolizes this seductive permissiveness of the analytic situation; and the switchman who is calling attention to the open door is the analyst. When the watchman asks whether the door was closed he is asking about this permissiveness of the analytic situation. "Were you not forbidden to take those pencils?" is the meaning of his question; and the patient answers "No," putting the blame on the analyst.

However, in the actual therapeutic situation the patient is not sure of the analyst's permissiveness. We suggested a moment ago that the watchman might be a projected image of the patient's conscience; but the dreamer's actual situation suggests a simpler explanation, that both the switchman and the watchman represent the analyst who, in spite of her seeming permissiveness, is also a forbidding mother figure to him. Although she seems to be encouraging his forbidden wishes, she might be offended as his mother would have been.

This conflict situation is the immediately effective stimulus for this dream. By comparing it with the dream text we can deduce what features of this stimulus situation are most disturbing to the dreamer and how he would wish to correct them.

(1) The dream text pictures temptation as occurring not in the analyst's office but in the freight yards where he works. Actually the patient is consulting the analyst as a physician; his relationship to her is a professional one. To protect himself from temptation he needs to reassure himself that the situation is really a professional one, not a personal relationship with sexual implications. The dream work has tried to carry this reassurance

further, substituting his relationship to the men on the job for his too personal relationship to the analyst. A number of references in dream text and associations emphasize this substitution of the less conflictful job situation.

(2) To protect him from temptation from a woman, the dream work has substituted two men. For his sexual impulse toward her, the dream has substituted a rather trivial symbolic act of stealing pencils from a boxcar.

(3) In reality the woman who is tempting him is the same one whom he is afraid of offending. To relieve him of this embarrassment the dream work has assigned the analyst's two conflicting roles to two different substitutes. By this device the dreamer is able first to respond to the temptation and then to deal with his fear of offending a parental figure. In this way the dream permits him to avoid confronting the two sides of his conflict.

VI

Following Freud we usually think that the dream censorship is exercised by the Superego. Yet it is evident from our analysis, that this dream's distortion of its picture of the conflict situation has not been motivated by guilt. The distortion in this dream is not a reaction of the dreamer's conscience to a forbidden wish. On the contrary, his guilt and his fear of offending the analyst are part of the conflict situation that has served as the dream stimulus. It is not only the forbidden impulse but the conflict situation as a whole that has been given distorted representation in the dream text.

To understand the motive and mechanism of the distortion in this dream we must reconstruct the problem which the dreamer's integrative mechanism faces. The patient's conflict in real life, which we have just reconstructed, is too great to be spanned by his integrative mechanism. It presents an integrative task that is in excess of his integrative capacity. In order to bring the dreamer's problem within the span of his integrative capacity the dream work has substituted an analogous but less disturbing problem. Similarly in waking life, when a problem is too complex to be grasped all at once, we may try first to solve an analogous but simpler problem.* Or, if one is too much involved in a controversy in actual life, it is often wise to withdraw to a distance for a time in order to view the points at issue with better perspective.

For our understanding of this device it is important to recognize that one cannot get rid of a disturbing conflict. For example, this dream could not wish its problem away; all that the dream work could achieve was to substitute a less disturbing but analogous hypothetical problem. And even this device gave only temporary relief; for the dreamer soon awoke with an acute attack of asthmatic wheezing.

VII

One of Freud's earliest insights was his discovery that hysterical symptoms are reminiscences; a hysterical symptom is the precipitate of a traumatic memory. His reconstruction of the origin of the conscience follows the same pattern: The conscience is a precipitate of the Oedipus complex. The normal conscience results from resolution of the Oedipus complex. An unresolved Oedipus complex leaves a neurosis or a neurotic character as its residue.

The Oedipus complex is, of course, not the only traumatic memory that can leave its traces in a patient's character. Even the dream that we have just been discussing involves a conflict that differs considerably from Freud's classical picture of a little boy's competition with the father for the mother.

From our analysis it appears that it is not his conscience but the analyst that this patient is afraid of offending. He reminds us of Anna Freud's child analysands. He has not yet acquired a Superego that is independent of support from a parental figure. He has not yet introjected parental prohibitions and imposed them on himself. He is much more afraid of a mother's disapproval than of his own conscience.

On the other hand, the inhibiting motive in this dream is not simply fear of loss of love. The watchman, when he appears, is not immediately offended but asks the patient to justify himself.

---

* For example, this is a technique frequently used in the solution of difficult mathematical problems.

The need to justify one's self implies a rule of conduct acknowledged by both accuser and accused. The rule of conduct to
which appeal is here made is one that is familiar in the nursery:
"Don't take things without permission." The patient's reply to
the watchman's question is a kind of shamefaced admission that
he has taken the analyst's permissiveness too seriously. However,
in the end the dream's attempt to justify him fails; for he awakens
wheezing with asthma.

When we transpose this scene back into the patient's childhood
it is evident that this little boy was too afraid of offending his
mother to come into active competition with his father. If our
reconstruction of this dream is correct, he has fled from a too
ambivalently personal relationship to a woman to a less threatening comradery with the men on the job; and when the watchman
appears it is not as a dreaded rival but as one who comes to en-
force the mother's authority.

The phantasied episode with the two men on the job is also
patterned on a familiar scene in the nursery—one in which a little
boy and his brother are caught by a parent in some trivial forbidden act. And the substitution of two men on the job for the
analyst suggests a pattern that may well have become established
in childhood—a pattern of turning for companionship to brother
or father figures when his relationship to his mother became too
conflictful.

VIII

And now, from this example, we can see the essential error in
our structural approach to the analysis of behavior. When we
read the Superego and the Ego into our analysis of a patient's behavior, we are trying to force the reactions of a particular individual into the pattern of a life history described by Freud as
typical. But no individual is entirely typical. Instead of using
Freud's account of the Oedipus complex as a Procrustean bed
into which everything must fit, we should try rather to find the
actual memories which have shaped the patterns of this particular
patient's behavior.

Thus we return to the method that was always basic in Freud's
attempts to interpret the neuroses. We search in our patient's

thoughts and behavior for the *persistent dynamic effect of particular traumatic memories.* Now that we are interested in the personality as a whole we modify this basic method of Freud's only by one slight shift of emphasis for which he has already shown us the way. We must now pay attention to both sides of our patient's conflict and try to reconstruct the problem with which the integrative mechanism is struggling. When we have once succeeded in reconstructing the patient's integrative problem and the integrative mechanism's method of handling it, we can often recognize easily the situations in the past that have patterned his behavior.

REFERENCES

1. ALEXANDER, FRANZ, M.D.: *Roots of Crime.* A. Knopf, New York, 1935.
2. ALEXANDER, FRANZ, M.D.: The Relation of Inferiority Feelings to Guilt. *Int. J. Psychoanal.,* 19:41, 1938.
3. FRENCH, THOMAS M., ALEXANDER, FRANZ, *et al.*: *Psychogenic Factors in Bronchial Asthma.* Parts I and II. *Psychosom. Med. Monographs* 1: no. 4, 1941, and 2: nos. 1 and 2, 1941. National Research Council, Washington, D. C.
4. FREUD, A.: *Introduction to the Technic of Child Analysis.* New York, Nervous and Mental Disease Publ. Co., 1928.
5. FREUD, S.: *The Interpretation of Dreams.* New York, Macmillan, 1913. Also in: *Basic Writings,* Book II, The Modern Library, New York, 1938.
6. FREUD, S.: *On Narcissim—An Introduction.* In: *Collected Papers,* Vol. IV. Third Edition. London, Hogarth Press, 1946, p. 30.
7. FREUD, S.: *The Ego and The Id.* Fourth Edition. Hogarth Press, London, 1947.
8. PIERS, G.: *Guilt and Shame* (To be published).

XI

THE INFLUENCE OF SOCIAL SCIENCE ON PSYCHIATRY

By

CHARLES S. JOHNSON*

It is attributed to Freud that he freed psychiatry from its rather rigid medical presuppositions, introducing a new and valuable interpretive psychology. There is an interesting area of speculation regarding the further and recent development of psychiatry, if Freud, in his personal background, had been as richly endowed in social experience as apparently he was in medicine and in classicism. For so much of what the social scientist regards as figurative expression, mechanistic determinism, symbolic interpretations, and individualism in his fundamental assumptions, seems to take human nature and culture into account, very largely as he functioned in it, incidentally, as a very special person, or as something with which the individual was in conflict.

When the late Dr. Harry Stack Sullivan described psychiatry as having to do with "interpersonal relations," a new dimension was added, and by a curious coincidence, the social psychologists noted that their field had shifted its center of gravity from concern with specific items of behavior and attitude to dynamic situational contexts, also involving interpersonal relations.

The farthest point reached with respect to mutual recognition by the respective disciplines, stemming from distinctly different origins, appears in a present preoccupation of the Group for the Advancement of Psychiatry, so well interpreted by Dr. Helen McLean in the statement:

"Over 50 years of investigation have made it clear that the total

_____
* President, Fisk University, Nashville, Tennessee.

personality of any human being is a socio-psycho-biological complex. The complexity of inter-relationships between forces in personality and forces in the environment is so great as to be almost beyond comprehension. The number of variables is staggering. The scientists' task is made more difficult by the added effect of one group on another. For full understanding there must be cooperative investigation by men in the psycho-biological sciences, and men in the social sciences, particularly, sociology and anthropology."

There is recognition by our leading sociologists and anthropologists of the contributions of psychiatry and psycho-analytical theory to the social sciences.

Professor E. W. Burgess notes the utilization of certain of the concepts in terms of social processes, in attempts at integration of viewpoints, concepts, and in a few cases, research methods. Freud's most valuable contributions to sociology, in his judgment, are the establishment of the role of unconscious factors in human behavior, emphasis on the role of wish fulfilment, and the analysis of the formation of dynamic traits and patterns in personality development independent of cultural influences. Some of the psychoanalytic concepts have been taken over suggestively and reinterpreted by the sociologists. The familiar term, "inferiority feelings," or "inferiority complex," is used by the sociologist to define a group attitude. *Resistance* is used to define the inhibitions imposed on individuals and groups by certain familial and cultural backgrounds and attitudes. *Mental conflict* is more often, for the sociologist, referred to a person involved in conflicting cultural elements of his society.

Kimball Young, another sociologist who has employed psychoanalytic conceptions and methods in a systematic way, finds the most significant contributions of Freud and his fellow workers to be first, the exposure of the importance of the unconscious motives and unconscious mechanisms in adult attitudes and behavior; second, the demonstration of the importance of the early years in laying the foundation of adult patterns, or life organization; and third, the emphasizing of the importance of the relations of the infant and young child to other persons, especially to members of his own family.

The cultural anthropologists have learned with the help of the psychiatrists, that the strictly social and cultural determinants, which, as Edward Sapir described it, give visible form and meaning, in a cultural sense, to each of the thousands of modalities of experience, could not possibly define the fundamental structure of a personality. It is clear that with the broadening of the concerns of both psychiatry and the social sciences, this area of exploration has found them increasingly on common ground. However particularistic the work of the psychiatrist, or however exclusive his preoccupation with the individual personality, there are common areas with the social sciences, as, for example, in the family matrix, which is a long established area of the social sciences. As Dr. Jules Henry of Washington University points out, ignorance of what goes on in the home of a patient is one of the banes of psychiatric therapy. To get the best picture of what goes on in the home, one would turn to the cultural anthropologist whose methodology in working with living cultures provides skills in direct observation of life as a basis for interpretation. At least such knowledge can sensitize psychiatrists to the problems involved. It is difficult to distinguish between what is purely cultural and what is purely interpersonal in mental problems. There are other common areas, such as delinquency, race, or other group prejudices, and even education. There is, in fact, in terms of developmental theory, an essential analogy between the growth of the individual and the growth of the group.

It might be well to consider for a moment, the factor of race prejudice in the etiology of the mental disorder of Negroes. Henry Myers and Leon Yochelson in reporting on a hospital service of nearly a thousand male Negro psychotic patients, were surprised to find in a large number of such cases, delusional material involving denial of color and ancestry. Most of the factual structure pointing to the influence of the complex race system on the picture presented by Negro psychotics is sociological, and, presumably, such knowledge is important to any effective treatment of the cases. What is involved is the structure and operation of the race system, variously in different areas, with definite limitations to status imposed by birth; the nature and function of stereotypes, color attitudes, the stock of ideas about race, patterns of accommodative behavior, color distinctions within the Negro community, social stratification, color symbolisms in the white and Negro communities, the social escape devices of avoidance, and "passing."

In 1940 Dr. Sullivan, who had developed a conceptual formulation of the relationship of the individual and the group, associated himself in the role of a psychiatric consultant, with a sociological study of Southern rural Negro youth.   In early recognition of the importance of cultural factors in the definition of personality, one of the basic challenges to this association sprang from an hypothesis regarding the effects upon personality of certain cultural patternings.   Sociological studies of the Negro in the South had suggested the existence, for historical reasons, of a strong matriarchal dominance in the rural or plantation Negro family structure.   If such existed there could be posed an interesting problem for the psychiatrist who had also made observations in China, where the family structure was decidedly patriarchal.

His memorandum on his psychiatric reconnaissance yielded observations more conspicuously related to the race system and the value systems of the dual societies than to the matriarchal hypothesis, and much, if not most of the working material for psychiatric interpretation came from the accumulated and organized knowledge about the social setting.   It would have been of little value three hundred miles North of the setting.   What he observed was an almost ubiquitous fear of white people, inter-racial attitudes, intra-group competition for personal advantages within the racial dependency relationship, illiteracy, low economic status adding to insecurity, stereotypes, hostility based on racial resentment of discrimination, social taboos, a rigid racial etiquette, anxieties, religious beliefs, racial ritual, "a timeless, formless optimism about life," and a cultural gap between himself and the plantation Negro that he could not bridge.

His conclusion was that "psychiatry, as the study of inter-personal relations has a difficult but a most rewarding field in the American Negro, that the Negro of the deep South seems in many respects the most promising for a beginning, and that he and his social situation, with its chronologically well-separated variations from the influx of new elements, constitute one of the most significant social science research fields."

It is, thus, not too presumptuous to list several types of conceptual and methodological influences of social science on psychiatry.

> (1) *The acceptance of the role of culture by psychiatry in the interpretation of the individual personality, and interpersonal relations, has made the psychoanalytic approach more compatible with the modern social-psychological approach.*

Psychiatrists appear to have recognized and adopted the concepts of society and culture for the richer and more realistic analysis of personality that they make possible. Sapir called attention to the close relationship of personal habit systems to the general patterning of culture. In a world of variant cultures and in societies with mixed and sometimes confused cross cultural relationships, the assumption of "universal feelings and attitudes" sentiments about parents, etc., is out of the question. This notion of the relativity of custom has long been one of the established assumptions of social science and, in particular, anthropology. It has been useful to psychiatry in providing a basis for the philosophy of behavior.

Karen Horney is an outstanding example of the growing number of psychiatrists who recognize the role of culture in personality formation. She recognizes that "abnormality" is relative to the culture in which it appears. In her view, society is not the enemy of the individual but something in which he participates. Her interpretations are essentially social-psychological in nature, and this may be said of many of the "Neo-Freudians."

> (2) *Acceptance of the sociological conception of "human nature" has modified some of the fundamental assumptions of psychiatry.*

Both psychiatry and sociology have shared the basic assumption that man is not born human. They have differed, however, in their conception of the manner in which man obtains the distinctive qualities of human nature. Following Freud, the earlier psychiatric assumption was that the human personality was a more or less abnormal or super-venient by-product of non-social, or even anti-social, instinctual tendencies. Sociologists, on the other hand, following the lead of Cooley, Dewey and others tended to minimize the role of instincts in human behavior. Writing of the supposed gregarious instinct Cooley said, "This is an easy, dogmatic way of explaining phenomena whose causes and effects are far more complicated than these others would admit. It seems to me to be the postulate of an individualistic psychology in search of one special motive to explain collective behavior. If you regard human nature as primarily social you need no such special motive."

Regarding human nature as a product of group life, Cooley stated: "It is the nature which is developed and expressed in these simple, face-to-face groups that are somewhat alike in all societies; groups of the family, the playground, and the neighborhood...In these, everywhere, human nature comes into existence. Man does not have it at birth; he cannot acquire it except through fellowship, and it decays in isolation." Sociologists, notably Ellsworth Faris and L. L. Bernard, took the lead in attacking the fallacy of explaining by "instincts" what was obviously habitual and customary behavior. Their strong challenge of the theory of instincts as significant motivations of human behavior brought a critical reexamination of the implications of instinct psychology by its psychoanalytic and psychiatric exponents. An increasing number of psychiatrists are now interested in obtaining and utilizing an accurate picture of the social realities by which the patient is surrounded, including the nature of the patient's participation in group life. The focus of psychiatry has been enlarged to view the patient not only as an individual body but also as a component part of a group.

(3) *The sociological theory of role-taking has been suggested as useful in defining the psychopathic personality.*

It is almost a truism that many psychiatric entities are to a large extent dependent upon sociological manifestations for their detection and definition. The definition of schizophrenia, for example, involves inappropriate social behavior, while the definition of paranoia involves the progressive misdefinition of social situations. Some sociologists have suggested that the sociological theory of role-taking may prove useful in understanding the psychopathic personality. That part of the personality which links an individual to the social community, often referred to as the "self," is a product of social interaction. According to George Herbert Mead, the self has its origin in communication and in taking the role of the other. Role-taking, or putting one's self in another's position, enables a person to predict the other's behavior. Role-taking ability makes one sensitive in advance to reactions of others, and provides a technique for self-understanding and self-control. The psychopathic personality may be described as pathologically deficient in role-taking abilities. Deficiency in role-taking means the incapacity to identify with another's point of view. The psychopath is unable to foresee the consequences of his own acts, especially their social implications, because he does not know how to judge his own behavior from another's point of view. The psychopath does not show intra-psychic conflict, or self-ambivalence, as does the neurotic and does not ordinarily seek counseling or therapy. He is not at odds with himself; he is at odds with the group because he is deficient in the capacity to evaluate objectively his own behavior against the standards of the group. The sociological concept of role-taking appears to synthesize a wide range of diagnostic and therapeutic data relative to psychopathy.

(4) *The growing psychiatric concern with the relationship of "social role" to personality development may be attributed to the influence of the social sciences.*

Any attempt to study social phenomena must make use of a definition of personality which emphasizes its orientation to social participation. The functions of personality are oriented in two directions: toward the internal process of the organism, and toward the social environment. There is continuous interplay between the relations of personality with the self, and relations with others. The concept of "social role" has been suggested as a bridge between the processes of intrapsychic life and those of social participation. Sociologists and anthropologists have used this term in various ways, but they have both tended, in common with psychiatry, to involve the elements of adaptation to social expectations as defined by social groups, especially the primary groups. The acceptance of this principle by psychiatry has tended to divert psychiatry from its former one-sided emphasis on the state of opposition between individual and society. Psychiatrists have come to recognize that under certain conditions, the forces of society and the individual may be antithetical; under changed conditions, these same forces may mutually complement one another. The concept of "social role" implies the capacity of the personality, in varying measure, to make fluid changes in form in accordance with the adaptational requirements of the individual's position in society. In a given time and social situation, certain components of the "total self" are mobilized into action, while other components are temporarily subordinated. With a change in time and group situation, a shift of "social role" occurs; that is, other components of the self are moved into a dominant position in preparation for a particular type of social participation.

This is the essence of the process of social adaptation. In this process, the individual may react to social pressure with compliance, protest, or withdrawal. There is also a fourth possibility, and this added possibility suggests a new explanation for war neurosis and psychosomatic disorders. If the social pressures are overwhelming or exceed the individual's resources for plastic adaptation, the organism may respond by disintegrating its old form and structuring a new form with distinct properties of its own. This is what seems to happen in psychotic forms of integration, in some forms of war neurosis, and in psychosomatic disorders.

(5) *The social sciences have furnished the foundation which enabled psychiatry to link medicine with the social situation within the broad context of culture.*

Psychosomatic medicine began initially with the recognition that environmental pressures which were contemporary and external to the individual might foster pathological conditions which affected the functioning of the human body. While this was a dramatic change from the older conception of the body as a mere collection of organs and faculties, it still left culture outside the individual. It has been relatively easy to identify contributing conditions in the immediate physical and contemporary environment with pathological conditions. The newer psychosomatic approach recognizes that the functioning of every part of the human body is moulded by the culture within which the individual has been reared. This includes not only diet, sunlight, and exposure to disease, but also the methods of rearing, punishing, and rewarding sanctioned by the society. The question may be appropriately raised that if an understanding of culture is essential to the understanding of the individual psychosomatic situation, how has the psychomatic approach been able to make such progress as it has without this essential element in its working hypotheses. In suggesting an answer to this question, Margaret Mead gives an interesting illustration and states that:

"because the physician is a member of the culture himself, he has taken the culture into account, only he has identified the particular type of cultural moulding which he sees in himself, his colleagues, and his patients, as human nature. It is as if a special kind of delivery with high forceps, which resulted in a distinctive moulding of the neonate's head, had become a universal obstetrical pattern in our society and all infants were delivered in this manner. Every physician who examined the head of a two-day-old infant would take this moulding into account in making diagnoses and prognoses. It is only necessary to forget or not to know that infants were ever delivered without resulting head moulding, for head moulding to be regarded as the inevitable effect of human birth. For practical purposes, the physician would make allowance for the head moulding, and it would not matter very much whether he regarded head moulding as the inseparable accompaniment of human birth, or as a mere item of cultural behavior, local in time and place. When, however, the physician, in addition to being a leader, is also a scientist interested in systematizing his knowledge of human heads and the significance of deviations in the shape of the head at two days old, then it would be absolutely essential that he should realize that this head moulding, which he always encountered, was something imposed upon the human organism by agents of the culture into which it was born and not the inevitable result of its humanity. So the psychiatrist, the psychoanalyst, and the wise physician have always operated with a working knowledge of our culturally standardized character structure, and called it 'human nature.' But the physician, qua research worker, needs to include in his conceptual scheme a recognition that man's biological potentialities can only be inferred from a study of human beings who have been subjected to many kinds of cultural pressures, and that no human being's behavior can be referred directly to these potentialities."

Such a recognition not only holds profound significance for preventive medicine, but for education and social planning generally.

(6) *Methodologically, the social sciences have influenced psychiatry by focusing attention on the value to be derived from direct observation of the total social situation of the patient.*

Harold Lasswell, in assessing the contribution of Freud to the social sciences, stated that he regarded the observational standpoint as exemplified in the insight interview as Freud's most abiding contribution to the social sciences. The psychoanalytic standpoint as developed by Freud was an interview rather than a participant, or spectator relationship. Lasswell compares the interview relationship favorably with each of the other three types of relationships. The "life-history" method of the social scientists reflects the influence of Freud's insight interview in a modified form. More recently, however, psychiatrists as well as others have pointed to the need for more direct observation of the total situation. William Healy, for example, expressing the point of view that there was a tendency to overvaluation of psychoanalytic concepts as providing solutions for many individual and social ills, he said: "Nearly all behavior problems are such because of their social significance. Conduct in general has positive or negative social values, and the problems we deal with clinically are of the latter type—ranging from those which merely cause annoyance to those which precipitate a demand for the protection of society."

Dr. Jules Henry of the Washington University Child Guidance Clinic, speaking of the orthodox psychiatric interview, says, "We have the description of the father in many cases only from the mother, or from the child. Our knowledge, if it may indeed be called knowledge, of the home life comes from an afflicted person. What we need...is a body of eye-witness accounts of what actually transpires in the home situation."

Mirra Komarovsky and Willard Waller have commented as follows in this connection: "Curiously, the parent-child relationship has rarely been studied from the point of view of the parent. Our knowledge of the relationship, though often profound, is therefore quite one-sided, and the advice which some of us rashly offer to the public is frequently impractical because it overlooks the parent and his needs." While pointing out that his suggestion of direct observation of the patient's social situation is a research proposal and not a continuing plan of treatment, Dr. Henry suggests that the cultural anthropologist and the psychiatrist would find value for both in working together even as a clinical team. Anthropologists and psychiatrists could both study the same mental cases, the therapist treating the patient and using the usual psychiatric techniques to concentrate on the psychodynamics of the individual case, while the anthropologist might study the cultural factors as expressed in the illness. Another form of cooperation between the two disciplines which might take place is through the formulation of hypotheses in regard to the essential core of specific syndrome types, which might then be studied cross-culturally.

   (7) *The social sciences and psychiatry have come more and more to share common areas of concern within the context of "personality and culture." This has resulted in psychoanalysts, anthropologists, and sociologists borrowing each other's knowledge and techniques.*

In the past few years, there have been purposeful attempts made toward the integration of viewpoints and concepts of psychoanalysis and sociology. This has been especially noteworthy in the area of family studies. Freudian psychology has been described in one instance, for example, as a sort of familistic social psychology which tends always to explain the behavior of the adult in terms of his previous experience in the parental family, frequently to the neglect of non-family and other later experiences.

Delinquency, race prejudice and education are other areas in which both the social sciences and psychiatry have worked. Although each discipline comes to the field with its unique standpoint and methods, the general impression is that psychiatry tends to assimilate the cultural referrents of social science more than the social sciences tend to assimilate the individual referrents of psychiatry.

It would not be appropriate to conclude this paper without stating that the contributions of psychiatry to the social sciences and of the social sciences to psychiatry are not universally acknowledged by the members of the two disciplines. The late Edwin H. Sutherland, writing in 1945, stated for example with respect to his field of interest that the psychiatric interpretations of criminal behavior, alcoholism, drug addiction, and other behavior patterns generally included in the field of social pathology are not sufficiently specific and definitive to be useful for sociology. Ellsworth Faris, while ackowledging the technique of "free association" as a distinct psychoanalytic contribution, proceeded to state that psychiatric presuppositions have often been uncritical and nearer intuition than science. Another facet of the problem was revealed in a symposium on *Methodological Problems in the Study of Social Phenomena* held at the annual meeting of the American Psychoanalytic Association in 1948. Some analysts were of the conviction that psychoanalytic study of individuals might provide considerable insight into the phenomenon of "social role," whereas others were doubtful and tended to reject the study of social phenomena as not belonging to the sphere of the psychoanalyst's everyday work with individual persons. Sapir himself stressed what he regarded as the fundamental divergence of spirit between the psychiatric and the strictly cultural modes of observation. In explanation of this he said, "I have done so because it is highly important that we do not delude ourselves into believing that a lovingly complete analysis of a given culture is *ipso facto* a contribution to the science of human behavior. It is, of course, an invaluable guide to the potentialities of choice and rejection in the lives of individuals, and such knowledge should arm one against foolish expectancies. No psychiatrist can afford to think that love is made in exactly the same way in all the corners of the globe, yet he would be too docile a convert to anthropology if he allowed himself to be persuaded that that fact made any special difference for the primary differentiation of personality." Kimball Young has stated this problem in more general terms: ". . . The Freudians have raised the basic problem whether there are not certain universal psychological mechanisms and patterns of child-parent relations which play a large part in personality development everywhere—that is, relatively independently of specific cultural training. While the culture will provide the framework for directionality and expression of these features, may it not well be that underlying the particular culturalized manifestations there exist basic social psychological factors common to all societies and their cultures? This is a key problem which neither cultural anthropology nor social psychology has as yet completely answered."

The need for a broad theoretical frame of reference for the integration of the manifold aspects of human nature and behavior into a unified picture of a man has led some social scientists and psychiatrists to call for a new science of personality. Dr. Andras Angyal, Resident Director of Research, Worcester State Hospital of Massachusetts, states that psychiatry is the application of a basic science which does not as yet exist. It is his contention that this basic science must be an entirely new science and not a mere combination of the results of physiology, psychology, anthropology.

The necessity and possibility of such basic science may be open to question, but should it be achieved it appears to be quite clear that its foundation would be found in the social sciences and psychiatry. If this be admitted, the urgent need is for a closer rapprochement between psychiatry and the social sciences. A synthesis of the contribution and of the methods of the basic life-sciences is needed. Their fruitful interaction will inevitably result in the beneficial integration of knowledge which marks the progress of scientific undertaking.

XII

THE THERAPEUTIC APPLICATIONS
OF PSYCHOANALYSIS
By
FRANZ ALEXANDER*

Psychotherapy as a systematic procedure practiced by medical specialists and based on a theory of personality is one of the youngest branches of medical practice. Psychotherapy as a practical aid given to a suffering human being is as old as any other method in the healing profession. Encouragement and consolation of the sick is an intrinsic part of every medical service. Even the most detached modern specialist who likes to think of himself more as an engineer or a glorified repairman rather than a healer, who treats his patient more as a defective machine rather than a suffering person, cannot avoid rendering, even unwittingly, psychotherapy. The patient will interpret his cool and detached attitude as the sign of the specialist's knowing what he is doing, and will extract from this some reassurance.

The elusive emotional component of the doctor-patient relationship has long been recognized; its therapeutic significance, however, was evaluated differently in the several periods of medical history. Only two generations ago the great clinician was proud not only of his wide knowledge of medical science [this was taken for granted] but particularly of his art of healing, the magical influence of his personality and his diagnostic intuition which he acquired through vast clinical experience. This stands in sharp contrast with the ideal of the modern clinician, whose forte consists in his highly technical knowledge of facts and pro-

* Director, Chicago Institute for Psychoanalysis; Clinical Professor of Psychiatry, College of Medicine, University of Illinois.

cedures. He acts almost as an industrial executive who receives
the results of various laboratory tests and the anamnestic history
from his interns, residents and subaltern associates and pieces together the diagnosis even if necessary without seeing the patient
longer than a few minutes. As Stephen Zweig so aptly stated:
"Disease meant now no longer what happens to the whole man but
what happens to his organs.... And so the natural and original
mission of the physician, the approach to disease as a whole
changes into the smaller task of localizing the ailment and identifying it and ascribing it to an already specified group of diseases.
...This unavoidable objectification and technicalization of therapy in the nineteenth century came to an extreme excess between
the physician and the patient became interpolated a third entirely
mechanical thing, the apparatus. The penetrating, creative synthesizing grasp of the born physician became less and less necessary for diagnosis...."

It is only recently that the pendulum of medical history began
to swing back again towards an interest in the patient as a person.
In the laboratory era the *thesis* was that the diseased body is like
a defective physio-chemical machine, and that healing consists
in repairing it by the methods of physics and chemistry. The
antithesis followed after the turn of the century—the claim that a
person is an entity, the whole function of which can be understood only in terms of psychology. Accordingly, the chronic
ailments of the body are merely the end results of the disordered
functioning of the main coordinator of the organism which we call
the personality. Etiological treatment must be directed ultimately to cure the disharmony in personality function by the
methods of psychology. This was the era which a great German
clinician called "Psychologismus in der Medicin." This attitude
is well illustrated by a cartoon reproduced recently in Leon Saul's
book, *The Bases of Human Behavior*, showing a physician who
assures his patient by saying, "Nothing is wrong with you. It
is all in your body."

Looking back upon these developments we may say now that
in the last two decades we are entering a new era of synthesis,
the psychosomatic era. This consists in the synthesis of the

thesis and the antithesis of the last half century, in the coordination and integration of the rich exploits of the laboratory methods with those of medical psychology. The initiation of this new Psychosomatic Institute of the Michael Reese Hospital is a living document of this historical process of integration by which the two main streams of modern medical progress—the physio-chemical and the psychological advancements—are becoming consistently interrelated parts of medical procedures. It is in this historical perspective that I shall approach the topic of my own presentation, the problems of psychotherapy.

It is not my aim to go into a detailed classification of the various psychotherapeutic procedures, and I shall deal only with the fundamental principles which serve as the basis of all sound psychological methods of treatment. Those who like clear-cut classifications and sharp distinctions between classical psychoanalysis, psychoanalytically oriented psychotherapy, brief therapy based on psychoanalytic concepts, will find my presentation unsatisfactory. They may even blame me for adding more to the already existing confusion instead of clearing it up. I am aware that with my treatment of this still controversial field I am incurring the danger of arousing the indignation of those who insist upon perpetuation of the existing sharp professional subclassification of psychiatrists into subspecialties according to the special techniques which they predominantly use in their therapy. I do not deny the practical inevitability of such specializations, as for example the practice of intensive reconstructive therapy in chronic neuroses by psychoanalysis which is so different from the custodial care of psychotics and from group therapy and even from the brief supportive treatment of acute cases. My belief is, however, that all forms of psychotherapy must be based on a thorough mastery of all the available knowledge—theoretical and practical—concerning the function and dysfunction of the personality. This knowledge —which is psychoanalysis—must be made available without distinction and discrimination to all those residents in the field of medicine who are going to devote themselves to the practice of psychiatry. Moreover, because the personality of the patient is a constant and significant factor in all diseases, a basic knowledge

of personality development and psychodynamics and principles
of psychotherapy must be an indispensable part of undergraduate
medical training.

After having thus defined my stand in regard to the position
of psychotherapy in general and psychoanalysis in special in the
fields of psychiatry and medicine, I shall attempt to formulate
those basic facts and assumptions which appear to me largely
uncontroversial and therefore suitable to serve as the basis for
all sound psychotherapeutic procedures. As I go along I shall
state my own position in regard to a few significant controversial
issues concerning the theory and practice of psychoanalytic
therapy proper.

In all fields of medicine the ultimate aim of treatment is to
eliminate the causes of disease and not merely the symptoms.
Merely empirical procedures, no matter how effective, are justly
regarded as less satisfactory. They are limited in their use and
incapable of methodical improvement, since the basis of their
effectiveness is not understood. Also, psychotherapy, as soon as
it claims to be considered an etiological treatment, must be
founded upon the knowledge of the disease process which it attempts to remedy. These are, in the first place, the psychoneuroses and all disturbances of the vegetative functions in which
psychological factors are of etiological significance. In all of
these conditions we deal with an impaired function of the ego.
When we speak of the ego, we refer to the organ system, whose
anatomical and physiological substratum is the highest integrative
center of the cerebrospinal nervous system. The function of the
ego consists in finding ways and means for the gratification of the
subjective needs by adequate behavior. In the ego's functions
three kinds of activities can be distinguished: (1) perception—
both internal perception of the subjective needs and the external
perception of the environment; (2) reasoning, which consists in
the integration of the data derived from both kinds of perceptive
activities; (3) the executive function which, based on the ego's
control over voluntary movements, consists in carrying out the
type of motor behavior by which the subjective needs can be gratified in harmony with each other and the existing external conditions. The fact that this complex three-fold function of the ego

can be disturbed in different ways accounts for the various types of mental disturbances.

One large group of diseases based on disturbed ego functions are psychiatric disturbances caused by organic changes of the brain tissue resulting from mechanical injuries or toxic influences or progressive degeneration due to the aging process. In such conditions psychotherapy has only an accessory and occasional application. In the advanced cases of major psychoses in which the disintegration of the structure of personality is excessive, yet no clearcut organic changes are demonstrable, the use of psychotherapeutic methods is still controversial. In most of these cases the constitutional factor, which is not accessible to psychotherapy, is of primary significance.

The principal field of psychotherapy is that group of psychiatric conditions which develop from injurious experiences in interpersonal relationships. These may be acute or chronic. In all these conditions, however, the paramount etiology consists in traumatic emotional experiences of the past; in the chronic cases mostly experiences of childhood, in the acute cases more recent adversities. Since the primary causes are emotional in nature, the appropriate therapeutic approach is also psychological.

I shall not undertake at this time the traditional way of presenting the principles of psychotherapy; namely, by reviewing its development. There are many excellent historical presentations of this field. I shall try this time to discuss the principles of psychotherapy from the point of view of our present-day knowledge.

ACUTE NEUROSES

Excessive emotions such as a paralyzing degree of anxiety, uncontrollable rage, continued relentless frustration, intolerable grief, may temporarily impair the ego's integrative and executive functions. The paralyzing effect of anxiety in an overwhelming startle situation is a common experience of everyday life and particularly of war. Also, excessive rage may narrow down the total grasp of the situation because an enraged person is apt to focus his attention on one single aim—that of vengeance, and disregard all other considerations. In general, one may say that in excessive emotional states the sole objective is to find immediate relief from the tension. This condition does not allow that amount of detachment which is necessary for the ego to have a comprehensive view of all the external and internal factors involved.

Well-known examples of acute neuroses are the different forms of war neuroses. But also in peacetime acute disturbances are not infrequent. They may assume almost any form—acute depression, anxiety states, hysterical conversion symptoms, vegetative disturbances of the visceral organs. These may develop in otherwise well-adjusted persons when exposed to life situations beyond their capacity to master. In the so-called traumatic neurosis, one of the important factors is the suddenness and the excessiveness of the trauma. In ordinary peacetime conditions in our so-called civilized existence, intricate interpersonal situations are the common causes. In such acute conditions it is obvious that the primary aim of therapy consists in reducing the intensity of the anxiety and the disturbing emotions by what is ordinarily called emotional support. The ego's functional capacity is fundamentally intact and is only temporarily impaired. Supportive psychotherapy may advantageously be combined with the administration of sedatives. Both the psychological support and the pharmacological effect of the depressants together contribute in reducing the intensity of the emotional tension and thus restore the temporarily disturbed capacity of the ego. The support consists primarily in talking over in a detached fashion the external situation, but may also include the clarification of some of the patient's emotional entanglements. The significance of such supportive measures should not be underestimated.

Acute neurotic disturbances, if not treated, can easily become chronic because the failure to meet an actual life situation may have in itself a demoralizing effect favoring the everpresent regressive tendencies of the ego. In its flight from the unsolved actual situation, the ego may return to poorly resolved conflict situations of the past which have some resemblance to the present conditions. Once the ego fails in its coordinating function in one situation, different kinds of mastery may break down. This explains why in traumatic neurosis the patient may lose such fundamental faculties as walking, speaking, in fact all coordinated movements, and may regress, although temporarily, to the completely helpless state of infancy. One must remember that a regressive tendency is present in everyone. Life under the best conditions is an arduous task. The universal need for periodic regressive evasion of the continuous stress of adjusted behavior is well demonstrated by the rhythm of life itself in the daily recurring need for sleep. Sleep can be considered as a physiological regression, and it demonstrates the need for a periodic recovery from stress through regression. When life conditions become difficult, the tendency to evade them by returning to the less responsible, more simple and more dependent situation of childhood is strengthened. Such a regressive evasion of existing difficulties is an integral part of every neurosis and psychosis whether chronic or acute. It is not quite inaccurate to say that in psychosis the person indulges permanently in a dreamlike state. All this explains why it is so important that acute conditions should be treated early, as Grinker and Spiegel have so ably demonstrated in their study of war neuroses. By helping to meet acute distress we help to restore the self-confidence and courage which are needed for the ego to make new attempts at tackling the pressing problems of life. Thus we prevent a further breakdown of the integrative functions, and deeper regression.

The same principle, however, prevails for all acute incipient neuroses of peacetime. The advancements in medicine in almost every field consists in the early discovery and treatment of incipient cases. The same is true in the field of psychiatry. The etiological understanding of neuroses as well as improved diagnostic facilities have changed the scope of psychiatry in a revolutionary fashion. While not long ago psychiatry consisted almost exclusively in the custodial care of advanced cases, modern psychiatric progress more and more takes place in ambulatory office practice. And in office practice the trend continues to be in the same direction. The practice of psychoanalysis some 30 years ago consisted primarily in treatment of the scarcely reversible cases of severe chronic neurotics. Psychoanalysis was the last resource and the psychoanalyst saw mostly the hopeless cases. Today with the public's becoming more psychiatry conscious, he sees more and more of the incipient cases where therapy has its greatest chances. This change in the patient material has required changes in psychoanalytic technique, which originally was worked out and adjusted to the needs of the most severe cases of neurotic disorders. The great variety of patients requires more flexible·technical applications of the basic therapeutic principles. To this many psychoanalysts responded at first with an unyielding insistence upon the classical procedures. They rejected the suggestions for modifications with the slogan that they are superficial. They saw any modification as a threat to the profundity and exclusiveness of psychoanalysis. They could not deny the need for a greater variety of analytical techniques and tried to save the day by declaring that anything short of the classical procedure should not be called psychoanalysis. This controversial issue is still not settled, but with the increasing recognition of the need for a greater variety of technical procedures based on the same scientific principles, the issue became chiefly a semantic one. No matter what these variations in technique are called— psychoanalysis or psychoanalytically oriented psychotherapy— the important fact is that they all require the same knowledge and training. Indeed, many analysts claim today that the flexible application of analytic knowledge requires greater experience and skill. This claim is justified because the practice of a routine technique does not require the same amount of judgment. It protects the practitioner from the arduous task of thinking and using his own judgment. So much about the treatment of acute and incipient cases.

CHRONIC NEUROSES

The chronic failures of the ego's functions develop gradually under the persistent influences of injurious interpersonal relationships. In most cases the disturbing experiences start in early childhood. When the traumatic personal relationships are of later origin and the early phases of ego development were sound, the neurotic disturbances resemble more the acute cases of later life. In chronic cases, merely supportive therapy is of little value, and the so-called uncovering types of psychotherapy are indicated. Since essentially all uncovering types of psychotherapy, no matter what name we attach to them, are based on the discoveries of Freudian psychoanalysis, we shall limit our discussion to the

principles of psychoanalytic therapy. These principles are valid
for the classical as well as for modified procedures.

The essence of psychoanalytic therapy consists in exposing the
ego in the treatment situation to the original emotional conflicts
which it could not resolve in the past. This revival of the pathogenic emotional experience takes place in the patient's emotional
reactions to the analyst, and is called the transference neurosis.
It consists in an irrational emotional involvement of the patient
with the therapist to whom he attributes the role of important
persons in his past life. The original neurotic conflict which consisted once in a disturbed relationship of the child to his family
environment now appears in a disturbed relationship of the
patient to the analyst. The irrationality of this emotional
involvement stems from the fact that the responses had sense only
in the past situation, and now they are repeated in the therapeutic
situation without the analyst's giving any provocation. This revival of the original conflict in the transference situation gives the
ego a new opportunity to grapple with the unresolved conflicts of
the past. Of course, the totality of the past situations cannot
always be revived in the transference. Experience shows, however, that the central dynamic axis of the old interpersonal conflict situation is always repeated in the transference situation.
According to this view, the fundamental therapeutic factor consists in that transference experience which is suitable to undo the
pathogenic experience of the past. In order to give the new
experience such a corrective value, it must take place under certain highly specific conditions. How to establish these conditions
is the main technical problem of the psychoanalytic treatment.

In exceptional cases an appropriate corrective emotional experience in the transference of sufficient intensity may alone
suffice to achieve far-reaching therapeutic effect. In most cases,
however, therapy consists of a series of consecutive and ever-
changing corrective emotional experiences, the corrective effect
of which depends to a large degree upon simultaneous insight. In
other words, in most cases the re-experiencing of the injurious
interpersonal relationship under the more favorable conditions
of the transference situation alone is not sufficient. The patient
must also obtain an intellectual grasp and recognize the past

sense and the present incongruity of his habitual emotional patterns. The relationship of emotional experience and intellectual grasp is probably the most difficult and most controversial part of psychoanalytic treatment. I shall try to indicate at least the most important problems involved without trying to give a final answer.

The first thing one must realize is that the new settlement of an old unresolved conflict in the transference situation becomes possible not only because the intensity of the transference conflict is less than that of the original conflict—as Freud expressed it, the transference is only a shadow-play of the original conflict— but also because the therapist's actual response to the patient's emotional expressions is quite different from the original treatment of the child by the parents. The therapist's attitude is understanding but at the same time emotionally detached. His attitude is that of a physician who wants to help the patient. He does not react to the patient's expression of hostility either by retaliation, reproach or signs of being hurt. Neither does he gratify the patient's regressive infantile claims for help and reassurance. He treats the patient as an adult in need of help, but this help consists merely in giving the patient the opportunity to understand better his own problems. He does not assume the role of an adviser nor does he assume practical responsibility for the patient's actual doings. He does not give the patient opportunity for any realistic blame or gratitude for anything but rendering a professional service. In the objective atmosphere of positive helpful interest the patient becomes capable of expressing his originally repressed tendencies more frankly. At the same time, he can recognize also that his reactions are out-of-date and are no longer adequate responses to his present life conditions or to the therapeutic situation. Once, of course, in the past they were adequate or at least unavoidable reactions—the reactions of a child to the existing parental attitude. The fact that the patient continues to act and feel according to out-dated earlier patterns whereas the therapist's reactions conform to the actual therapeutic situation makes the transference behavior a kind of one-sided shadow boxing. He has the opportunity not only to understand his neurotic patterns, but at the same time to experience intensively the irrationality of his own emotional reactions. The fact that the therapist's reaction is different from that of the parent to whose behavior the child adjusted himself as well as he could with his own neurotic reactions makes it necessary for the patient to abandon and correct these old emotional patterns. After all, this is precisely the ego's function—adjustment to the existing external conditions. As soon as the old neurotic patterns are revived and brought into the realm of consciousness, the ego has the opportunity to readjust them to the changed conditions. This is the essence of the corrective influence of those series of experiences which constitute the transference.

In this discussion one basic fact has been simply stated and no attempt made to explain it. I refer to the fact that the patient in the objective, encouraging attitudes of the analytical situation spontaneously expresses his basic neurotic patterns in relationship to the analyst, or in other words, that he will develop that transitory artificial neurosis which Freud called the transference neurosis. Time does not allow me to go into a detailed discussion of why and how the transference neurosis unavoidably develops in all cases of chronic psychoneurosis if the analyst's attitude is appropriate. It might suffice to state that the analytic situation encourages a temporary regression to infantile attitudes because all evaluative reactions on the analyst's part are consistently absent. It is under the normative influence of the parents that the inhibitions and repressions developed. Neurotic patterns are nothing but maladaptations to the standards which the parents represent. In most cases they can be traced to more intensive repressions than is common in normal people. These old behavior patterns become conserved because their exclusion from consciousness does not allow their continuous adaptive modification which is required for normal development during emotional maturation. Neurotic symptoms are a combination of substitutive outlets for asocial impulses and at the same time defenses, such as denials, compensations and self-punitive reactions to these original non-social impulses. As Freud said, the neurotic is at the same time more and less social than the healthy individual. He is more social inasmuch as he is more inhibited, has more intensive guilt feelings, is more self-critical and self-punitive than a normal. Yet at the same time, he is less social because his symptoms or his neurotic acting out are substitutive expressions of unadjusted impulses. In many cases a fascinating and intricate interplay of extremely primitive impulses with overly social, often self-punitive, self-destructive responses can be observed. The permissiveness and the lack of evaluations in the psychoanalytic situation has a tendency to counteract repression and mobilize the original impulses which were repressed under the influence of parental intimidations. Thus a freer expression of the original neurotic patterns is encouraged. This process is complicated by the fact that much of the original parental-child relationship has become internalized in the case of chronic neurosis. The external struggle between child and parents, the expression of hostility and sexual impulses, of guilt, expiation by suffering and punishment—all this complex interplay between the child and his environment becomes transformed to an internal struggle. The parental images become incorporated as part of the personality in the form of the superego, and the external battlefield of emotional interplay becomes transplaced into the internal arena of the personality. The emotional interplay between the child and parents becomes an internal conflict between differentiated parts of the personality. During psychoanalytic treatment the intrapsychic conflict becomes again transformed back into its original interpersonal form as an interplay between the patient and the physician in the transference situation. Only after this externalization of the intra-psychic conflict has taken place and the transference neurosis has developed can the real therapeutic task be undertaken—the treatment and cure of the transference neurosis.

In this phase of the therapy which often takes place after a brief period of time, sometimes within a few days, sometimes several months of treatment, the analytic task becomes: (1) to keep the intensity of the emotional participation of the patient on an optimal intensity; (2) to give insight by interpretations; and (3) to create an emotional climate in the treatment situation which will favor the patient's need to correct his reaction patterns to the new interpersonal situation. The nature of this interpersonal rapport is what I refer to as the emotional climate of the treatment. It is in this phase of the analysis when the analyst's own attitude becomes of paramount importance. This brings us to another controversial and not yet fully explored problem of analytic treatment which is known as the problem of counter-transference.

The original concept of Freud was that the analyst functions as a blank screen upon which the patient projects his own subjective distortions. He attributes to the analyst the roles of the originally important persons of his past. In the patient's mind the analyst may become the intimidating or loving father, the rejecting or overprotecting mother, the rivalrous older brother or any important person whose influence has been preserved in his unconscious, and which is again revived in the transference. It is obvious that the more neutral the analyst's attitude is, the less will he interfere through his actual personality and actual behavior with the patient's tendency to attribute to the analyst whatever role suits his needs. Theoretically, this position is consistent, yet it does not precisely describe the phenomena which takes place in treatment. The analyst remains a real personality for the patient no matter how neutral he tries to be. As soon as the transference relationship is well established, the analyst's own spontaneous responses to the patient, often called countertransference, are of great significance in hastening or retarding the process of readjustment.

I should like to make this concrete by one example.

Let us consider one of the frequent occurrences in the transference. The patient repeats toward the analyst a combination of hostile rivalry and guilt which he entertained towards his father and which he never could resolve. Let us further assume that the original conflict developed because of the extremely permissive attitude of the father towards his son to whom he could not deny anything. This occurs often when the father identifies himself with the son to an excessive degree. His father might have treated him with lack of understanding and rejection. This made him so sensitive towards the helpless child that in order to save his son from the suffering to which he was subjected in his own childhood, he leans over backwards and tries to gratify all the son's wishes. Yet, in spite of his father's generosity, the son becomes involved in the oedipal rivalry with him because of his

strong attachment to his mother. As a result, an intensive conflict develops between hostile rivalrous tendencies toward the
father and his feeling of love, admiration and gratitude. This is
an impasse which is difficult to solve even for a fully mature
person. The child often succumbs to this emotional impasse and
chooses one of the many possible neurotic solutions. One of these
is to provoke the father into hostile behavior by irritating and
tantalizing him. Should he succeed in provoking the father to
express anger and hostility, he will be relieved from his guilt
feelings. Then he can feel hostile without intense conflict. With
an overly indulgent father such victories, however, are extremely
rare, and he will have to repress not only every aggressive impulse but every other form of self-assertion. Such a patient in
the transference situation after the transference neurosis has developed will attempt to repeat the same behavior formula toward
the analyst. He will develop toward him a hostile competitive
attitude which will take some specific form depending upon the
actual life situation. He will envy the analyst's success and will
resent the analyst's position of authority. At the same time, he
will feel the same guilt towards the analyst who tries to help him.
If the analyst's attitude is sufficiently neutral, the patient will
attribute to him the role of the father. As the treatment pro-
gresses and the defenses are reduced, the patient's hostility will
be mobilized. The problem of countertransference must be considered at this point.

The analyst remains a person in his own right. The blank
screen is an abstraction which does not correspond exactly to
reality. The analyst has his own emotional reactions toward the
patient whether he expresses them overtly or not, and it is not
easy to conceal them without special effort. These emotional
reactions are determined by his own past history. He may react
to the patient's rivalry and provocation with some resentment.
Another analyst may be unaffected by this and will react more as
the patient's own father did, with indulgence and sympathy.
Then the patient will face the same situation he faced in his
childhood. Since his guilt does not elicit any reprisals from the
analyst, his own guilt feelings will mount and require further repression of every aggression. He may continue for a while with

his attempts to elicit some sign of rejection on the analyst's part. After a while the situation may become intolerable, and he must either leave the analyst and find a less sympathetic one or repeat his own neurotic adjustment to the indulgent father figure—inhibition and turning his hostility against himself in the form of depression. It is obvious that the more the analyst's unconscious countertransference attitude which, of course, in a well-trained analyst will never find drastic expression, resembles that of the patient's father, the less chance there is that the patient will feel the need to correct his own pattern. He can well utilize his own neurotic pattern, which is nothing but an adaptation to the pattern of overindulgence.

Recently many analysts have become interested in this elusive phenomenon of countertransference. It has become a particular issue in the training of analytic therapists in the so-called supervised analyses. In observing the student's attitude towards the patient many teachers have discovered that quite often the analytic process becomes stymied on account of the inexperienced student's lack of ability to control his spontaneous countertransference attitudes. If the countertransference attitude happens to be the same as the original parental attitude, the patient will have no difficulty in repeating his original father-son conflict in the transference situation, but it will become extremely difficult for him to modify it.

Let us return to our example. Let us assume now that the analyst does not react with such indulgence to the patient's provocations. He may even knowingly, or unwittingly, express some kind of resentment and rejection of the patient. This is a novel situation for the patient, whose old pattern does not fit. He finally succeeds in provoking the father image and therefore his own guilt for his hostility will decrease. Now he can express his hostility toward the analyst. The defense mechanism has broken down. In certain patients such an expression of hostility might mean an unavoidable transitory step toward achieving a full mastery over hostile impulses, not by repression, but by achieving conscious control.

In a difficult treatment of a neurotic young man of this type many years ago, an inadvertent expression of my resentment against the patient's provocative attitude had an unexpected therapeutic result. Some months previously the same patient left his former analyst who carefully avoided expressing any displeasure with the patient's extremely provocative behavior. He behaved exactly as the patient's father did. No matter how precise his interpretations were, his attitude created an intolerable emotional paralysis in the patient—a complete inability to express any self-assertion and to tolerate any success. He not only did not improve, but became even more inhibited and depressed. Finally he left the analyst, accusing him of insincerity. The inadvertent expression of some resentment on my part provoked an initial perturbance after which the patient's behavior underwent a rapid change. He discovered that not everybody was like his father, and in order to be liked and accepted by others he had to make himself acceptable by them. At the same time, the need to expiate his guilt, which had become so intolerable on account of the limitless indulgence of the father, became less necessary for him, and therefore he could give up his continuous need for failure and could accept success without internal remorse.

At that time, I had already come to the conclusion that, once the transference is well established, and at the same time the analyst has understood the pathogenic situations of the past, the analyst may do more than control his own countertransference reactions and try to be the blank screen of Freud's. At the beginning of the treatment, to be sure, such a neutral attitude is necessary in order not to interfere with the development of the transference neurosis. But once the transference relationship is well established, certain countertransference reactions will develop in the analyst as a response to the patient's transference. He must not only recognize and control these countertransference attitudes, but he can advantageously replace them with a type of response which is suitable to call for readjustment on the patient's part. Occasionally, his spontaneous countertransference attitude may be helpful by chance. For example, in our case, in this phase of the treatment the analyst should make the patient feel that his provocative behavior will make it much more difficult for the analyst to like the patient, but nevertheless, being a doctor he will not cease to try to help him. Yet, the analyst should certainly not respond in such instance to the patient's provocation with extreme indulgence. Without intimidating the patient, at the proper time of the treatment the analyst may display a reasonable amount of displeasure. The patient will thereby find it easier to resolve his original conflict which became so intolerable because of the father's unlimited indulgence. The display of some displeasure is particularly important in such a case as this, because the patient can easily misinterpret the analyst's patience and helpfulness as overindulgence. In my case the expression of displeasure on the part of the analyst had a double effect; it reduced the need for self-directed aggression, but it also demonstrated the undesirable consequences of the patient's provocative behavior. This does not require, however, a violent dramatic explosion on the part of the analyst. It suffices that he lends to the analytic situation an emotional climate to which the patient's neurotic problem does not fit. He will then be compelled to find some new way to resolve his conflict.

The intuitive analyst will often act just in the described manner. Our aim is, however, to replace intuition with conscious understanding. No matter how one feels about the use of planned therapeutic attitudes, one thing seems to be incontroversial; namely, that the spontaneous countertransference attitude might be helpful in one case, but unfavorable in another. Therefore, there is no doubt that the analyst's awareness of his actually existing and spontaneous emotional reactions to the patient and a conscious control of them means a distinct and important advancement in the field of psychoanalytic therapy. It is early to predict how much not only a conscious control but utilization of countertransference attitudes or their replacement by planfully adopted emotional climates of treatment will increase the effectiveness of psychoanalytic therapy. One must remember in this respect that when Freud originally discovered the phenomenon of transference, he considered it as a particular complication of the therapeutic process which in those days he conceived primarily as an intellectual process of self-understanding. We know today that the transference which was once regarded as an impurity has become the axis of therapy. It is not impossible that the new impurity which we have discovered—the analyst's response to the transference situation—may become in the future an equally important dynamic instrument of psychoanalysis.

In the foregoing discussion we have focussed our attention primarily on the technical significance of the emotional experiences which take place during analytic treatment. In emphasizing these emotional aspects, we must not forget the significance of intellectual insight. We must remember that a neurosis consists in impairment of the ego's integrative and executive function. Both of these functions are based on insight or in other words in the intellectual grasp of the internal needs and the existing conditions in the environment upon which the satisfaction of the subjective needs depends. In neurosis this integrative function of the ego is impaired. According to the original concept of Freud, the weak ego of the child in order to defend itself against alien impulses and emotional constellations which it could not handle in the past has to exclude them from the realm of consciousness. These defenses become automatic, the psychological meaning of which is excluded from the realm of the ego. It has lost control over them. During psychoanalytic treatment we try to re-expose the ego to that which it has repressed in the past. This requires the overcoming of those resistances by which the ego defends itself against this unbearable psychological emotional content. As we have seen, the most important factor in overcoming the resistances consists in a nonevaluating attitude of the therapist because the parental evaluations are at the basis of most repressions. In addition to this emotional factor we must consider also intellectual insight. Intellectual insight means mastery. It is the forerunner of control. Inasmuch as insight increases the ego's mastery, it decreases its anxiety from the repressed content. Intellectual understanding obtained by interpretative work as a rule is the precursor of emotional experience of repressed content. By intellectual insight the ego is, so to speak, prepared for what will appear in the consciousness and is not taken unawares by a sudden break-through of terrifying unconscious material.

In this light psychoanalytic therapy appears as a complex, slowly progressing interplay between intellectual insight and emotional experience in which old interpersonal relationships, internalized and buried in the unconscious as intra-psychic conflicts, become revived again as external conflicts between the patient and the analyst. In this way, both intellectual understanding of the conflict situation and the correction of rigid automatic neurotic patterns become possible. Psychoanalytic treatment is neither an emotional gymnastics alone nor a merely intellectual process, but a delicate combination of the two. The analyst's role, accordingly, is a complex one. He becomes in a sense the target of the patient's neurotic reactions, and at the same time also an interpreter, who aids the intellectual integration of the uncovered material which the patient dramatically expresses in the transference.

The combination of emotional experience and understanding can take place in many variations of treatment procedures. The treatment may consist in daily interviews continued over years; it may be a considerably briefer procedure. I cannot at this time go into all the technical details, particularly not into all the suggestions concerning the time factor. The more we understand the fundamental processes which underlie the psychoanalytic process, the more we can emancipate ourselves from routines and habits which tend to formalize analytic treatment and to make it less effective.

I cannot leave this topic, however, without referring at least briefly to one of the central difficulties of prolonged psychoanalytic treatment. This is the occasional extreme prolongation of the treatment. I cannot refrain from saying that this fundamental difficulty has not been faced by us in the past with the courage necessary to deal with it. We fell into the habit of dissipating our concern for the excessively long duration of some treatments by not always valid excuses. We say that if the so-called period of working through is handled with sufficient patience and tenacity, eventually even an unusually prolonged treatment can be successfully terminated. Unfortunately, this is not always the case. Or we declare the patient is incurable. The problem of interminable cases is, indeed, a serious one. Are these cases all really incurable, and must psychoanalytic treatment in such patients be considered as a life-long crutch? Or is in many cases the prolongation of the treatment due to a lack of full understanding of the quantitative aspects of our procedure? Freud discovered this central problem of psychoanalytic treatment rather early in his career. He discussed it in one of his articles on technique. He said that his initial difficulty was to help his patients to remain under treatment; later he encountered the opposite difficulty, namely, that his patients' desire to recover became outweighed by their desire to be treated.

With this statement Freud recognized one of the fundamental problems of psychoanalytic treatment. In the light of our present theory this difficulty is easily understood. We know that the patient sooner or later will replace his original neurosis with the transference neurosis in which intra-psychic unsolvable conflict situations are reconverted into interpersonal neurotic reactions between the patient and the physician, which are replicas of his early neurotic involvements in the family. This transformation contains elements of gratification for the patient. He is allowed to keep his neurosis as a necessary part of the treatment. Both he and the analyst encourage each other that this neurotic personal relationship will end sometime in the indefinite future. This offers an extremely seductive alibi for the patient to continue to be neurotic and for the analyst to continue to treat him. The patient can retain gratification of his dependent needs which cause less and less conflict in the permissive and understanding atmosphere of the analytic situation. At the same time, he saves face by assuring himself that eventually he will be cured by continuing the treatment. In many cases if the patient can financially afford it and the analyst feels that he gets sufficient intellectual rewards from the treatment, this becomes an impasse. The transference gradually loses the feature of suffering which to a high degree derives from the intra-psychic nature of the original neurosis, and now the condition is reached in which the wish to retain the dependent relations to the analyst will outweigh the wish for recovery.

After years of experimentation many of us in the Chicago Institute became aware of the necessity to combat from the beginning of the treatment the regressive-dependent component of the transference situation. No matter how valuable and indispensable a factor it may be, it must be kept on an optimal level by making it conscious and keeping it conscious. This can be done only by frustrating it. The most powerful frustration consists in well-timed reductions of the frequency of the psychoanalytic interviews and well-timed shorter or longer interruptions. Routine continuation of the treatment in daily interviews over years may favor the regressive tendencies to such a degree that some patients will never be able to renounce them. We know well how difficult it is to take away gratification from a person to which he has acquired certain rights by habit and custom. The problem of how to handle the patient's dependent needs is a central issue of psychoanalytic therapy and it will remain in the future one of the most difficult technical issues. In order to cure the patient we have to allow him some regression to an infantile state. We have to make this regression even rather comfortable and relatively devoid of conflict. We pay for this powerful therapeutic device with the difficulty of terminating the treatment. All this amounts to the fact that the medicine of artificial regression in the transference can be given in overdoses. Like radiation therapy, it is a powerful weapon, but can become the source of a new illness. Like x-ray, the transference situation is also not an undangerous instrument. In order to improve the therapeutic procedure we must become aware not only of its beneficial aspects but also of its hidden dangers. There is no use in denying that together with its brilliant successes, the history of psychoanalysis is full of interminable patients. Not all of these cases are incurable, and we will be able to help them by learning how to administer in desirable quantities the most effective factor of psychoanalytic therapy—the revival of the infantile neurotic conflicts in the transference situation.

In recent years a division has become apparent in the still small community of psychoanalysts. On the one side there are those who feel more satisfied with our present knowledge and therapeutic techniques, who are apt to look suspiciously upon innovations, and who try, therefore, to preserve psychoanalysis in its original form. This attitude is opposed by those who are keenly aware of the gaps in our theoretical knowledge and of the weak spots in our therapeutic procedure. No matter which of these two attitudes is more valid, it is certain that the mere repetition of routine and the denunciation of every new suggestion as a threat to the purity of psychoanalysis can only lead to stagnation. Let me conclude by emphasizing that further improvements of our therapeutic methods can only result from a persistent re-examination of our theory and from relentless experimentation with technical modifications.

XIII

CRITIQUE OF SYMPOSIUM
By
JOHN P. SPIEGEL*

N° symposium is truly complete without a summation or analysis of its content. An inspection of the contributions to this symposium affords an illuminating review of the current phase in the development of psychiatry. The key to this phase is a steady expansion of the field of observation. The range of observations currently significant to psychiatry would have seemed fantastic fifty years ago for then the attention was fixed on psychopathology, and the morbid anatomy presumed to underlie it. But in the first year of the second half of the twentieth century this focus appears myopic. The concern of the psychiatric investigator and clinician has shifted and broadened from a virtually exclusive preoccupation with disease—at the psychological and biological level—to an interest in *health and disease* as varying aspects of the same underlying process of adjustment. The basic process is understood as the method whereby the human organism maintains itself in relatively stable equilibrium with its environment. Health and disease are distinguished from each other by virtue of the degree of success or failure of the adjustment process, but the sharpness of the distinction blurs as the observer scans the totality of human behavior.

The enlarged vista, however, is not completely accepted. The

---

* This critique was written by the Associate Director of the Institute for Psychosomatic and Psychiatric Research and Training after the entire symposium had been delivered. He had no part in choosing the constituent papers nor did he read any of them before delivery. Thus, after sitting through all sessions as an objective observer he was able after digestion of the material, to write this succinct and lucid critical summary.

general agreement that human behavior must be understood in its totality is accompanied by some truculence and skirmishing between the various cooperating parties. By and large there is a concensus regarding the three principle levels of abstraction from the totality of human behavior: biological, psychological, and social. It is understood that no discipline working at any of these three levels of abstraction, no matter how entrenched in tradition, can now remain aloof from the others. All are included in the common field of observation, the extended vista. But as the traditional boundaries melt away, some of the observers feel ill at ease with the new company in which they find themselves. The insecurity and anxiety become evident as a concern for orthodoxy and a resistance to change. Nevertheless, the effect on the whole is salutary and leads to an intense interest in collaboration between the disciplines.

Collaboration, however, is not possible without readjustment— an attempt to bring concepts stemming from the different disciplines into line with each other. Thus the neurophysiologist searches for keys with which to integrate his basic conceptual units, neurones and cortical architectonics, with the simplest psychological units such as gestalt mechanisms and conditioning. Whether concepts related to communication engineering and electrical and chemical field theory will accomplish this result remains to be seen. Similarly, the psychologist attempts to throw off his laboratory harness, to get rid of oversimplification and artificiality, and to study the healthy adjustments of human beings in various settings. The field approach in psychology, with its emphasis on mutual interactions between the human being and the environment in which he lives, seems particularly fitted to bring psychological concepts into line with participant-observer methods of psychiatry. From the opposite direction, the psychoanalyst struggles to shed his metapsychological shackles so that on the one hand he can integrate instinct theory with the physiological substratum from which it springs, and on the other build a bridge between his concepts of character structure and function and the cultural and family setting of which any character must be formed. The sociologist is a hardworking partner in the construction of this same bridge, and it seems quite likely that such concepts as social role, and the multiple facets of role-taking will prove highly useful building blocks.

All these efforts at collaboration lend an excitement and a ferment to the field of psychiatry which only partially conceal the existence of the basic, serious problem whose solution is necessary before a real consolidation of the current gains can take place. This problem is the lack of a conceptual scheme, pitched at a level of abstraction from human behavior appropriate to the unification of the various points of view. What exist currently are patchworks of concepts loosely basted together by naive operations which do not satisfactorily achieve multilevel correlations much less their integration. Undoubtedly there is virtue in the mere accumulation and matching of concepts derived from the various levels of abstraction. But this is only a beginning. Both the weakness and the strength of this symposium lie in the clarity with which it reveals the need for a methodological solution to the problem of the integration of the disciplines contributory to the science of human behavior.

XIV

CLOSURE

By

Roy R. Grinker

The Institute for Psychosomatic and Psychiatric Research and Training of the Michael Reese Hospital has on this day, June 1, 1951, arrived at a state of being. It has required long and careful planning by many persons who have been unswervingly loyal to the goal of comprehensive medicine. As at all births we have celebrated this event by a ritualized ceremony. Scientists have offered many words of wisdom concerning the achievements of ancestral disciplines and have forecast a wonderful future for the new edifice erected for the science of behavior. In symbolic manner we have eaten and drunk and enjoyed good fellowship.

But, I feel the need to close this celebration on a final serious note. Although our joy at the opening of the Institute and our gratitude to the community and those special persons who have given us this opportunity, is great, we have now assumed a tremendous responsibility. To plan and build the structure has required much work and great sacrifices, but there has always been the pleasure of envisaging the time when our goal would be reached. That has come to pass and everyone can see that the product of all our endeavors is beautiful—today. But, what will its development be? What will be its role in research, in education, in help for the sick? These questions can never be finally answered and our anxieties regarding them will be perpetual with no end-point, no goal to reach, no surcease from effort.

We could make firm resolutions tonight and glib promises for the future. However, in our present mood I think it better to express our credo in the form of fervent wishes somewhat in the

182

manner of prayerful hopes. With much help from many people some of these wishes may be gratified:

1. May our assumptions be undistorted and faithful to the proven labors of our scientific predecessors.
2. May the questions we ask of nature be reasonable and appropriate to the problems of unitary man.
3. May our powers of observation be sharp and our technique of measurement accurate.
4. May we have the breadth of knowledge to include in our study of behavior all possible help from the concepts, operational methods and knowledge of many disciplines of science.
5. May our emphasis on understanding human behavior not lead us to neglect any level of biological activity properly identified, nor confuse several levels in false correlations.
6. May we strive for originality, for freedom of imagination and for courage to leave the highway for new and un-broken paths toward our goals.
7. May we never become structuralized in our concepts, ritualized in our procedures or formalized in our therapies.
8. May we ever strive to transmit clearly without pride our knowledge, and with humility the fields of our ignorance to the eager, curious students of all fields.
9. May we strive to apply our learning to the preservation of health and the treatment of illness.
10. May the promise and hope of this Institute be transmitted without decrement to many generations of young, fresh and enthusiastic workers to whom we shall give unre-stricted opportunities for help and progress.

This Book

Mid-century Psychiatry

Edited by ROY R. GRINKER, M.D.

was set and printed by the Mack Printing Company of
Easton, Pennsylvania, and bound by Arnold's Book Bindery,
Reading, Pa. The engravings were made by the Capitol
Engraving Company of Springfield, Illinois. The page trim
size is 6 x 9 inches. The type page is 26 x 43 picas. The
type face is Linotype Caledonia set 11 point on 13 point.
The text paper is 70-lb. Warren's Olde Style. The cover
is Bancroft's Linen Finish 3390.

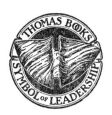

With THOMAS BOOKS careful attention is given to all
details of manufacturing and design. It is the Publisher's
desire to present books that are satisfactory as to their
physical qualities and artistic possibilities and appropriate
for their particular use. THOMAS BOOKS will be true to
those laws of quality that assure a good name and good will.